# LIVER DETOX & CLEANSE

## THE NATURAL WAY TO IMPROVING LIVER HEALTH

BRITTNEY DAVIS

CRAIG WILLIAMS

© Copyright 2020 - All rights reserved Admore Publishing

Paperback ISBN: 978-3-96772-027-3

Hardcover ISBN: 978-3-96772-028-0

The content contained within this book may not be reproduced, duplicated or transmitted without direct written permission from the author or the publisher.

Under no circumstances will any blame or legal responsibility be held against the publisher, or author, for any damages, reparation, or monetary loss due to the information contained within this book. Either directly or indirectly.

Cover Design by Rihan W. Cover artwork from DepositPhotos

The Icons used in this work were designed by:

- Kirill Kazachek, prettycons, Smashicons, Vitaly Gorbachev, surang, turkkub, Freepik, wanicon, and Eucalyp from Flaticon.com
- DepositPhotos

Published by Admore Publishing: Roßbachstraße, Berlin, Germany

Printed in the United States of America

www.publishing.admore-marketing.com

**Disclaimer**

This book contains collected information from top experts and sources. All details have been carefully researched and selected but are for informational purposes only. It is not intended to be interpreted as professional medical advice or replace consultation with health care professionals.

Speak to your trusted healthcare professional prior to undergoing any medical procedures, taking any nutritional supplements, or starting an exercise regimen. Reactions and results vary from each individual as there are differences in health conditions.

If you have any underlying health conditions, consult with an appropriately licensed healthcare professional before considering any guidance from this book.

## OTHER BOOKS BY BRITTNEY & CRAIG

- Gut Detox & Cleanse

To find more of our books, simply search or click our names on

www.amazon.com

# CONTENTS

| | |
|---|---|
| Foreword | ix |
| Introduction | xiii |

| | |
|---|---|
| 1. ALL THINGS LIVER | 1 |
| Locating Your Liver | 2 |
| Digestion and Absorption of Nutrients | 3 |
| Production of Proteins | 5 |
| Storing Nutrients | 6 |
| Hormone Production and Regulation | 6 |
| Excretion and Detoxing | 7 |
| Just All-Round Amazing | 8 |
| 2. COMMON LIVER DISORDERS, SYMPTOMS AND CAUSES | 11 |
| A Complex and Carefully Balanced System | 12 |
| *Hepatitis* | 13 |
| *Autoimmune Hepatitis* | 14 |
| *Primary Biliary Cholangitis* | 15 |
| *Primary Sclerosing Cholangitis* | 16 |
| *Hemochromatosis* | 17 |
| *Wilson's Disease* | 18 |
| *Alcohol-Related Liver Disease* | 19 |
| *Cirrhosis* | 20 |
| *Liver Cancer* | 21 |
| *Fatty Liver Disease* | 22 |
| *Non-Alcoholic Fatty Liver Disease* | 23 |
| Drug-Related Liver Disease | 24 |
| The Golden Rules of Liver Disease | 25 |
| 3. IMPROVING LIVER HEALTH | 29 |
| Simple Changes, Big Results | 30 |
| Nutrition and Your Liver | 31 |
| The Healthy Liver Diet | 42 |
| Drinks for Liver Health | 46 |
| Body and Soul | 47 |
| Things to Avoid | 50 |

| | |
|---|---:|
| Mental Health Issues | 52 |
| Review Prescriptions | 52 |
| Build Liver Detox into Your Life | 53 |
| Weight Loss and Liver Health | 54 |
| You are in the Driver's Seat | 55 |

## DETOX & CLEANSE

| | |
|---|---:|
| Detox & Cleanse | 61 |
| Breakfast | 65 |
| Lunch & Dinner | 87 |
| Snacks | 107 |
| Juices & Shakes | 109 |
| Juices & Shakes Continued | 115 |
| 7 Day Meal Plan | 117 |
| 7 Day Meal Plan Continued | 119 |
| 4. SHAKE WHAT YOUR MAMA GAVE YOU! | 121 |
| How Exercise Helps Your Liver | 122 |
| Yoga | 123 |
| Afterword | 133 |
| Thank You | 137 |
| Resources | 139 |
| Other Books By Brittney & Craig | 143 |

# FOREWORD

Hi there,

We are Brittney Davis and Craig Williams, and we are passionate about all things health and wellness. Our purpose is to help others in all aspects of building great habits and living a healthier, better life!

You may have grabbed this book because you are interested in finding out more about how the liver works.

Perhaps you are looking for specific guidance on how to best improve your liver health and so your overall health...

... Or you are simply on the look for some great meals and recipes that can help your body naturally detox.

*Whatever the reason,* **we want to thank you for reading and checking out this book.**

In this book, our aim is to provide a straight-to-the-point, scientifically accurate action plan to enhance liver health. Unlike other health books that focus on overhyped, unhealthy methods to potentially lose weight and detox, we hope to provide you with techniques to improve your wellbeing in a natural form.

Although it's great to read this book all the way through, feel free to skip ahead to different parts you are more interested in. We will cover various topics ranging from liver anatomy and liver diseases to natural detox recipes and health tips. Skip through topics that may not apply to you and get to the things that may be individually relevant to you!

We sincerely thank you again for your interest. Enjoy!

❝

It is health that is real wealth and not pieces of gold and silver.

---

*Mahatma Gandhi*

# INTRODUCTION

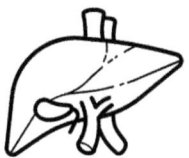

---

*Burnout:* - *"A syndrome resulting from chronic workplace stress that has not been successfully managed."*

---

Most of us have experienced symptoms of burnout. You constantly lack energy and feel exhausted throughout the day. Your body is present, but your mind wanders and dreams off, so your job, daily tasks, and loved ones suffer.

You aren't effective and are just mentally drained.

For many of us, our livers are suffering through this exact same process. It may surprise you, but this triangular-shaped 3.3-pound gland is largely responsible for keeping your body and mind functioning properly.

It is working 24/7, and although our bodies are amazingly efficient and designed perfectly... it is possible to hit a wall.

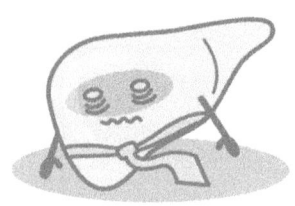

Unknowingly, many of our daily habits do a lot of harm to this vital organ.

Everything you drink, eat, and even place on your skin in terms of lotions and cleaning products get filtered or comes into contact with your liver.

When was the last time you gave any thought at all to your liver?

If you are like most people, you rarely think about it at all.

In fact, when most people think about improving their health, they think of losing weight, gaining muscle, and the newest diet trends.

Next, we worry about our appearance and inner health of our hearts, our brains, our lungs, and our waistlines. We obsess about wrinkles and examine food labels in microscopic detail. But, unless we have a specific reason to worry about our livers, we rarely give them a second thought.

That is a big mistake because the liver is one of the most important (albeit least "flashy") organs in the body. In fact, it has a key role to play in most of the things the better known, more highly regarded organs do.

It produces chemicals that are important for digestion and the excretion of harmful chemicals.

It manufactures several important hormones that help to keep our bodies in balance.

It converts excess glucose to glycogen for storage, and it produces several proteins that are essential to everything from transporting fats around the body, to producing plasma.

Without the liver, we would not be able to clean toxins out of our blood, regulate blood clotting or extract and store iron from hemoglobin.

In fact, medical experts have discovered that our livers perform over 500 functions essential to our health and well-being. Many of those are so critical you would not survive if they did not happen. So, you could say your liver is a sort of biological life support.

It is your largest internal organ, and it works quietly and tirelessly, 24 hours a day, seven days a week, every day of your life, keeping toxins at bay and helping to keep everything in balance.

It can heal itself over time, and it is the only organ that you can receive a partial transplant of, from a living donor, and regrow to its full size over time.

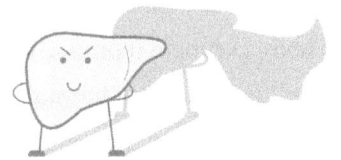

In short, it is a biological superhero, well hidden behind some nerdy spectacles, and its high time we paid it a little more attention.

But, because it is so important to literally everything that our body does, that also means that when things are not quite right with your liver, you might find that you experience some strange symptoms.

This book hopes to peel back the mask on your superhero liver, and help you understand how things like burnout, fatigue, unexplained abdominal pain and even itching and bruising could be a coded message from this important organ.

We will show you the things you might be doing that cause your liver to have to work harder, or worse, cause it damage. We will look at what happens when your liver is not working at its full potential, and what you can do to give it a helping hand.

Then we will show you how everything you eat, drink, and even put on your skin is eventually filtered through your liver. You will discover how the life you lead directly impacts your liver health – and how that can affect how you feel overall.

The good news is that one of the most amazing secrets locked in your liver is its remarkable ability to repair itself and regenerate. So even if you haven't been taking great care of yourself or your body, you can make changes today that will help your liver get back on track. Since it is involved in nearly everything your body does, this could be the start of a total body transformation.

What Is Your Liver Affecting?

You are going to read a lot more, in detail, about what your liver does and how it helps nearly every system in your body to function properly, and we're going to show you how to get it working optimally through simple lifestyle changes.

But before we get to that, you should know what less than fantastic liver health might be causing or exacerbating in your life right now.

You might be experiencing fatigue or burnout because your hormones are not balanced, or you are not using nutrients at peak performance. You may be experiencing appetite loss, or you might have metabolic issues that cause you to gain weight even when you control what you eat, or you might find that you bruise easily, or that your hair and nails do not grow as quickly as you would like them to.

All of these, and more, are things that could be directly related to your liver health.

## Why Read This Book?

Whether you are experiencing fatigue or burnout, loss of appetite, weight gain, or poor hair and nail growth, the solution may be improving liver health. If you are concerned about the above points, worried about liver disease, or are just looking for easy ways to improve your health and energy levels, this book **is for you**. It's also for anyone who wants to know how to take better care of their liver before they experience damage or injury and want to reap the benefits of more energy, better skin tone, and less bloating or swelling.

If you care about your health, then you need to care about liver health. We're going to tell you how everyone can make simple changes, starting today, that will keep this miraculous organ healthy. This will profoundly impact the way you feel, look, and experience every day of your life.

We will show you what you might be doing in your life that is placing undue strain on your liver, and what you can do to change those habits.

We'll teach you how to take better care of your liver so that you're working with this remarkable unsung health hero, and we'll give you recipes, tips, and more to make liver health part of your healthy living plan.

Improving liver health is an important step on your road to a better, healthier, more fulfilled life, but it doesn't have to be hard to do. Everyone can make small changes and see a BIG impact.

We cannot tell you whether your health problems are caused by your liver. Only your doctor can diagnose specific conditions and symptoms. But we can tell you that improving liver health will enhance everyone's overall health somehow and often very dramatically.

So, if you are looking for effective ways to make positive health changes in your life, it is guaranteed to have an impact.

Good health is not something you buy from the pharmacy. It is not something you get from a plastic surgeon, or by trying the latest diet trend. It is a collection of tiny steps that you repeat often enough that they become good habits. The more of those small steps you take, and continue taking, the more you will start to see visible results in your life.

## What This Book Is

After years of researching the root cause of problems like fatigue, burnout, feeling mentally drained and physically tired, we know that achieving better liver health will change your life. So, let me show you how you can as well, quickly, easily, and without expensive pills, magic health potions, or complicated routines.

Most of us don't realize the stress we place on our livers, and because it's such a durable organ, don't experience enough liver trouble to seek medical advice. These years of neglect add up and mean there is a high probability that many of us are suffering from the ill effects of not taking better care of our livers.

Even if you do not have a severe liver condition, you may still be doing incremental damage, and you may be feeling the effects of less than ideal liver function in your life. Over time, you may start to experience more severe effects, or you might just keep feeling like something is missing, not working properly, or just a little off.

This book is a science-based, easy to follow, no fluff guide to liver health. We are not going to try to sell you any "magical" liver products or a regime. We are not going to judge you for lifestyle choices or expect you to feel guilty for having a little fun from time to time. We do not expect you to spend a fortune on complicated therapies with little or no basis in science.

Good health doesn't have to be complicated or costly, so we just want to show you how you can do all those things, and still take care of your liver, so your liver can take care of you.

This book is a simple guide to what your liver is, what it does, why it might not be working to its peak potential, and what you can do to change that. It's about what your liver health might be affecting in your daily life, and what warning signs you might see.

So, if you are looking for a practical, no-nonsense approach to make a definite improvement to your health, this book is for you.

## What This Book Is Not

As much as we would love for it to be, unfortunately, this book is not going to be a magic cure for everything that ails you. If you have been experiencing specific or worrying symptoms, we strongly recommend that you consult your doctor as soon as possible, as you should in any medical situation. Books can educate and inform, but they cannot diagnose or treat, so do not take the risk if you think you need medical intervention!

This book is not a medical guide to the liver. It is a personal account of how we have researched the science of liver health and used it to improve our health, lives, and well-being.

This book is also not a quick fix. There is no miraculous potion that will give you immediate improved liver health. However, there are natural ways you can help your liver do its job better and more efficiently. There are no gimmicks, no pills that can erase bad choices overnight, and no shortcuts.

But if you are willing to put in a little work, make some manageable changes to your lifestyle, and listen to your body a little more... You can transform the way your liver works, and reap the benefits in nearly every aspect of your overall health.

Now that we know what this book is and is not, let's get down to business, and learn more about what your liver is, how it works, and what it does for you.

> 

If you have no time for Health, Health has no time for you.

*Justin Zheng Jixin*

# 1

## ALL THINGS LIVER

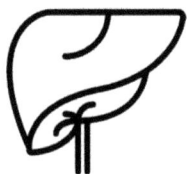

All of us are born with what can technically be considered a superpower.

Your liver is the only organ in your body that can completely regenerate and heal itself over time. In fact, because of this miraculous ability, the liver is also the only organ that can be partially transplanted from a living donor – and then both the donor and recipients liver will regrow to full size.

That's not all though, even if up to 75% of your liver were removed, the miraculous organ would regrow to be fully functional in just 10 days.

That's a good thing too, because while you can get dialysis for damaged kidneys or a pacemaker to correct the beating of your heart. There is still no widespread mechanical or technological support options for liver function.

Your liver is an amazing, miraculous, and hard-working organ, but the more you know about how it works, where it is, and what it does, the better you understand how to keep it healthy.

Locating Your Liver

Your liver is actually the largest internal organ in your body. It is about the size of a football, and it sits mostly in the upper right quadrant of your abdomen – between the diaphragm and the stomach.

Your liver is made up of two lobes, each of which are divided into eight segments. These segments are made up of thousands of small lobules, and all of those are connected by a vast network of ducts. All of those ducts are interconnected to form the common hepatic duct, which is the channel that transports bile out of the liver once it has finished its work of cleaning up toxins from your blood.

The liver also receives and transports blood by several major blood vessels, including the hepatic portal vein and the hepatic arteries.

Much of the liver's almost magical abilities is because of the incredibly unique type of cells it is made of. These cells, known as hepatocytes, make up about 80% of the liver by mass. They are the cells that synthesize and store proteins, transform carbohydrates for storage, detoxify, excrete and modify substances in the blood, and create cholesterol, bile, and other chemicals and compounds our bodies need to function.

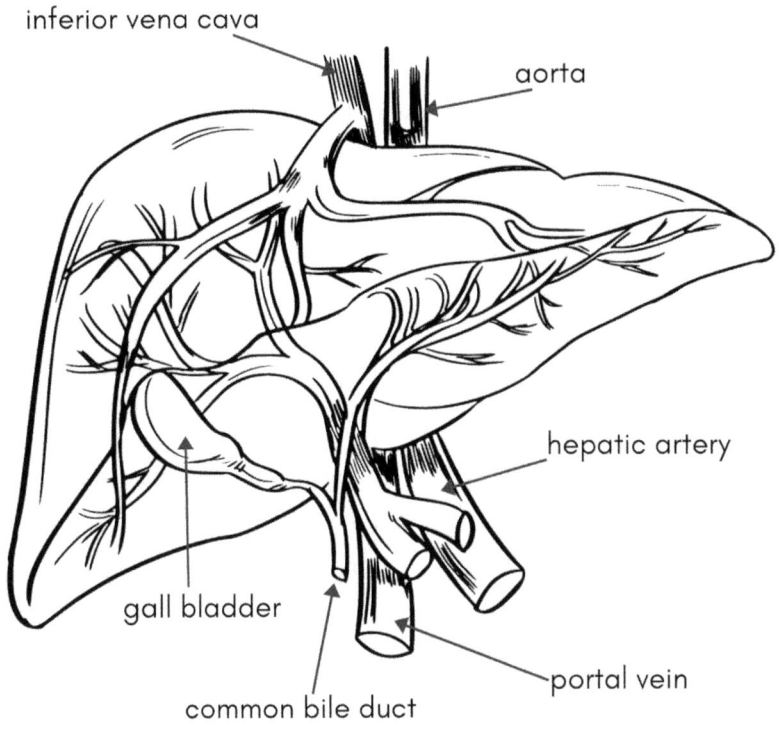

Since your liver does so many things for you, we thought that an excellent place to start would be to look at some of the more important functions this remarkable organ performs.

Digestion and Absorption of Nutrients

When you think of your digestive system, your liver probably is not the first thing that springs to mind. In fact, you might not even know that your liver is involved in the process. But, while your stomach and intestinal tract are the stars of this vital system, they would not be able to get the job done without your liver.

There are two ways that your liver helps your body make the most of the food you eat.

Firstly, it produces the chemicals that turn the nutrients you get from food into the compounds your body needs to function. Think of it as an organic factory, manufacturing finished products from raw materials. It is like an extremely complicated biological refinery. It takes your food from a crude state to highly specialized fuel to power your cells and keep you healthy and happy.

Secondly, it produces bile, which is essential in processing fats and certain nutrients.

In fact, without bile, you would not be able to process fat at all because it is bile that emulsifies the fat cells, and allows the small intestine to absorb them. Since vitamins D, E, K and A are also fat-soluble, if it were not for bile, you would not be able to absorb them.

Your liver takes over right at the end of the digestive process. Sorting the good stuff from the bad, and ensuring that the nutrients absorbed by your intestinal tract are transformed in the most efficient way possible.

Since the food we eat is fuel for our bodies, it is easy to see how if your liver is not functioning at its peak, you might have less energy and struggle to get through the day.

But it is also so much more... fats and oils, for instance, contain substances like Omega 3 fatty acids. Those are important to weight loss, brain function, preventing and reducing inflammation, and reducing insulin resistance, which is very important in Type 2 diabetics and prediabetic people.

If food can be seen as medicine, then your liver is your body's chemistry professor, transforming everything we eat into the perfect balance of substances to heal, support, and improve our health.

Production of Proteins

The chemical powerhouse that is your liver does not only turn the food you eat into the fuel your body needs. It also manufactures many important proteins that do all sorts of essential things in your body.

For instance, blood clotting would not be possible without your liver, which produces most of the coagulation factors your body uses to heal internal and external wounds.

Since the liver also produces albumin. Another protein that regulates blood volume and distribution of fluids in your body, it is intricately woven into the circulatory system and every other organ and system in your body.

You would not be able to store iron without your liver, either. It produces ferritin, which is the protein that helps to transport iron around your body. Since anemia often comes with chronic fatigue, it makes perfect sense that if yours is not working at its peak, you might be suffering from an iron deficiency.

Lipoproteins are another particular type of protein that is only produced in your liver. You might have guessed from the name that they are instrumental in the movement of cholesterol around your body, and as you probably know, cholesterol levels are critical to heart, vein, and artery health.

These are just a few of the particularly important proteins your marvelous liver quietly makes, helping to keep all the other chemicals you need and systems you rely on working properly.

Storing Nutrients

So far, we have only covered a small section of all this magnificent organ is capable of...

Your liver is also the critical link in storing and releasing a variety of nutrients you need. Excess energy from carbohydrates, for instance, is stored in your liver as glucose. It then works with your pancreas to determine when this stored energy needs to be released, to keep your body fueled and ready. This is another reason why, if your liver is not working optimally, you might find that you lack energy. If it is too busy taking care of other functions, it might not be releasing that stored energy when you need it!

Your liver stores and processes fats, produces and regulates cholesterol levels, and breaks proteins down into the amino acids your body needs to build new muscles and make important repairs.

In other words, your liver is one of the star players in your metabolic system, and when it is working correctly, it helps to ensure that everything stays in balance. This means if you are eating a healthy diet and exercising regularly, your liver helps to ensure that you stay in great shape and look great too!

Hormone Production and Regulation

Need another reason why your liver is a rock star? How about hormone production and regulation?

Your liver converts thyroid hormones into their most active form. Since your thyroid also plays a role in your metabolism, this makes your liver a double whammy in ensuring that you are processing the food you eat most efficiently.

It makes IGF-1, which promotes cell growth, and it also produces Angiotensinogen. This is a hormone that helps regulate sodium and potassium in the kidneys and helps keep your blood pressure stable.

But your liver does not stop at making these especially important biological chemicals. It also breaks them down and gets them out of your body when you have too much of them, helping to keep everything in the careful balance we need to be healthy.

Excretion and Detoxing

Last but certainly not least, your liver is the organ that is responsible for filtering toxins, neutralizing them, and getting them out of your body.

Your liver processes chemicals ranging from alcohol and drugs to excess biological chemicals out of your blood, rendering them harmless, and sending them on their way.

While this may not sound as exciting as regenerating or manufacturing proteins, if these chemicals were allowed to build up in your body, they would quickly become extremely dangerous. Eventually, the buildup would even become fatal.

By filtering an endless list of potentially dangerous chemicals, compounds, and proteins out of your blood, your liver is literally saving your life every day.

## Just All-Round Amazing

The truth is, your liver is simply amazing.

It is the most complex organ in your body, at least as far as the number of different processes it does for you goes! It contains over 300 billion specialized cells and those cells process over 1.7 liters of blood every minute! In fact, at any time of the day, your liver probably holds about 13% of your blood supply.

Your liver produces about a liter of bile per day, but it also processes and disposes of any you do not use. It holds enough vitamin A to keep you healthy for about two years.

If you are a woman and are planning to get pregnant (or already expecting), your liver is doing a lot of heavy lifting too! In fact, because your liver is essentially "working for two" while you are growing a baby, it can nearly double in size for expecting moms.

Without your liver, you would not be able to properly regulate your blood pressure, store energy, remove toxins from your blood, or regulate your metabolism. Your blood would not be able to clot, and you would either have too much or too little of it. You would not even be able to use many of the nutrients you eat, because there would be no way to transform them into usable chemicals.

There is simply no organ in your body that does as many things for as many systems and processes as your liver. This is why it is so vitally important that you take good care of it, so it can keep taking good care of you.

Now that we know what your liver does for you, it is time to learn what you can do for your liver.

> You can enhance your body's natural detoxification system by simply changing your diet.

*Women's Health Network*

# 2

# COMMON LIVER DISORDERS, SYMPTOMS AND CAUSES

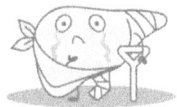

We now know that the liver can be pretty much looked at like your body's MVP. Like with every most valuable player, without it, the team that is you, would not get very far.

Nearly every process in your body depends on your liver at some point, and if you want to have a championship body, you need to learn how to take great care of that star player. One of the most important ways to do that is to learn more about what might go wrong with your liver, why it might happen, and the warning signs.

As with everything health-related, when something is not right with your liver, the sooner you act, the more likely you are to have a good result. Whether that means lifestyle changes or something else, learning to spot the common signs of liver trouble is essential to your overall health.

This chapter is all about the more common liver disorders out there, how you might spot the signs that you need to seek medical care, and what might happen if you are diagnosed with one of them.

## A Complex and Carefully Balanced System

Your liver is the engine that drives what is called the hepatic system. This is the system that, as we have already discussed, cleans your blood of toxins, helps you digest food, creates bile, and more.

We have also discussed how your liver is the most complex organ in your body, and that also means that it is carefully balanced. When an injury or illness throws that balance even a little off, you will notice signs that something is not right.

Before we get into the specifics of some of the things that might cause that, it's important to remember that if you have any medical symptoms or signs that something might not be right, you should consult your doctor.

There is a fair amount of stigma surrounding liver disease because most people believe that it is always related to alcohol or drug abuse, which is not true. Even if you are experiencing liver disease-related symptoms because of lifestyle choices, the best thing you can do for yourself is to seek help and make the necessary changes to improve your health.

Treating your liver right will have a profound change in your general health, and you owe it to yourself to find out what the cause of your symptoms is and get the right treatment.

Now that we have got that out of the way, here are some of the more common liver diseases and disorders you should be looking out for.

*Hepatitis*

Hepatitis is a blanket name for inflammation of the liver. This usually occurs due to the viruses known as Hepatitis A, B, C, D, and E, but can also be caused by lifestyle factors like excessive drinking. Some people also develop hepatitis as a result of autoimmune conditions or drug use, whether prescription or otherwise.

Some people also get Hepatitis C through sexual activity, so if you are sexually active, you may be at risk of contracting this version of the virus.

The symptoms of hepatitis can range from very mild and almost unnoticeable to very severe, including death. If it is chronic, or ongoing, rather than acute (sudden onset that resolves within weeks or months), hepatitis can also trigger more severe diseases like cirrhosis or liver cancer.

There are vaccinations for Hepatitis A, B, and D, but none for Hepatitis C. There are, however, antiviral medications and other treatments that can treat all kinds of hepatitis, which is why it is crucial to seek a diagnosis if you think you might be affected.

Hepatitis symptoms can range from almost none to a telltale yellowing of the skin, nausea and vomiting, other tummy trouble, fatigue, and abdominal pain. Any or all of these symptoms may also be accompanied by loss of appetite.

Diagnosing hepatitis can be a tricky process because it is not always caused by the same thing.

If you have yellow skin and eyes, your doctor will probably consider hepatitis right away. Still, in other cases, it may take a medical and travel history, blood tests, and different tests and processes to determine if your symptoms are caused by hepatitis – and which type!

It is always good to get vaccinated for the types of hepatitis that there are immunizations available for, especially if you travel a lot.

Treatment for hepatitis will also depend on the type you have. Your doctor may recommend bed rest, dietary changes, lifestyle changes, and medications. You will probably have to have regular checkups after diagnosis to make sure that things are progressing as desired.

Hepatitis can be dangerous and debilitating, and in some cases, the disease can be exceedingly difficult to beat. Still, if you seek help early, and listen to your doctor, most people can regain liver health over time.

### Autoimmune Hepatitis

We have briefly mentioned it before, but it deserves its own section as well.

While most types of hepatitis are caused by external factors (alcohol abuse or a virus), some people develop autoimmune hepatitis. In this case, their own body attacks their liver, causing damage and some potentially severe symptoms.

Like most autoimmune diseases, no one knows what causes autoimmune hepatitis. The symptoms are remarkably similar to other types of liver disease. They may include fluid in the abdomen, unexplained swelling of your limbs, and other, more severe problems.

People who have autoimmune hepatitis are usually treated by specialists called Hepatologists. Their treatment will typically include steroids and other drugs to suppress their immune system. In very severe cases, people who have autoimmune hepatitis may require a liver transplant.

## Primary Biliary Cholangitis

Primary Biliary Cholangitis or PBC used to be known as Primary Biliary Cirrhosis. Still, because cirrhosis is only a factor in very advanced stages of the disease, it was renamed to include milder forms too. PBC is an autoimmune disease that specifically affects the bile ducts. Like all autoimmune diseases, when you have PBC, your own body attacks itself, in this case, by destroying bile ducts.

This is an exceedingly rare condition, affecting about 1 in 4000 people. Still, of those affected, about 9 out of 10 are women, so it is far more likely to be the cause of your symptoms if you are a woman.

PBC has similar symptoms to other liver conditions at first, but as more and more bile ducts are destroyed, symptoms become much more pronounced.

If you suspect you may have an autoimmune liver disease like PBC, your doctor may use everything from liver enzyme tests to antibody tests, ultrasounds, and biopsies to confirm the condition.

Once confirmed, you will be treated with a combination of medications and lifestyle changes, which will likely include synthetic bile, supplements to compensate for poor absorption of vitamins and other nutrients, and drugs to control symptoms. Dietary changes and alcohol avoidance are also part of the treatment plan for people with PBC.

There is no cure for PBC, but treatment can control the symptoms. In severe or advanced cases, liver transplants can improve the quality of life for people with PBC.

*Primary Sclerosing Cholangitis*

Primary Sclerosing Cholangitis or PSC is another liver disease that most people have never heard of, but that may be behind common liver disease symptoms.

Unlike many liver ailments, however, PSC is often considered idiopathic, meaning that there is no definitive cause.

Some people believe that it is an autoimmune disease, but it does not respond to conventional autoimmune treatments like other diseases of the type.

Some studies have shown a connection between PSC and intestinal flora, while others link the condition to cellular senescence, which is a condition where cells effectively stop replicating.

There are also potential links to genetic factors.

However, with no concrete or definitive cause for PSC, it is awfully hard to say with any complete certainty what might trigger this condition. That also makes it a lot more complicated to treat this condition.

One of the main signs of PSC and one that your doctor will be on the lookout for is sclerosis of the bile ducts, which means that the ducts narrow and harden, and cannot perform their function at their peak. There are several tests that your doctor may use to confirm the diagnosis, including serum alkaline phosphatase (ALP), cholangiography, which is a "picture" of your liver that shows the narrowed ducts, and a liver biopsy.

There are no drugs specifically indicated for treating PSC, so your Hepatologist will work with you to find a treatment plan that helps you manage the disease and the symptoms. Because treatments are limited, people who have PSC are likely to require a liver transplant at some point.

## Hemochromatosis

Most of the diseases and conditions we have discussed so far have been acquired or later-onset conditions. However, there are also a few genetic or hereditary liver conditions that may cause trouble for your liver and your overall health.

The first one we want to discuss is called Hemochromatosis, and it is all about iron buildup in your body, and in particular, your liver.

We need iron to be healthy, but people who have Hemochromatosis absorb more iron than they need from the food they eat. Their bodies are unable to get rid of the excess iron in their blood. Low iron in the blood can cause a condition called anemia and be extremely dangerous, but too much iron is toxic, and can also be life-threatening if not treated.

Hemochromatosis is usually genetic, in which case it is called primary Hemochromatosis, and is one of the most common genetic conditions in the United States. In some cases, however, other diseases, liver damage, and alcohol use can trigger "secondary Hemochromatosis," which has the same symptoms but is not a congenital condition.

The prognosis for people who have Hemochromatosis depends on how early the condition is diagnosed. The longer it goes untreated, the more likely that there will be serious damage to several organs. This includes severe liver disease and even liver cancer, heart problems ranging from arrhythmia to heart failure, diabetes, arthritis, and various glandular conditions.

There are several treatment options your doctor may recommend if you have been diagnosed with Hemochromatosis. These may include dietary changes to cut out high iron foods and vitamin C (which can increase iron absorption), a medication-based treatment known as chelation, and therapeutic phlebotomy, a process where some of your blood is removed to lower your iron levels.

Your doctor may also need to treat secondary conditions that have been triggered by your Hemochromatosis diagnosis.

*Wilson's Disease*

Wilson's disease is another genetic condition that affects the liver, but in this case, instead of an accumulation of iron, your body builds up dangerous levels of copper.

Like iron and many other minerals and metals, your body needs a small amount of copper to maintain health, build and maintain your nervous system, bones, and skin. However, like any other metal, too much of a good thing can be life-threatening when it comes to your body, not filtering and removing enough of it.

People who have Wilson's Disease are born with the condition, and most are diagnosed sometime between 5 and 35 years old.

Symptoms are similar to many other liver conditions, including fatigue and jaundice, swelling or edema, and a lack of appetite. Some people will also have abdominal pain, and you may also have Kayser-Fleischer rings, which is a discoloration of the eye.

If you have these symptoms, and especially if you have a sibling or a parent diagnosed with Wilson's Disease, it is best to get diagnosed as soon as possible. The longer copper builds up in your liver, brain, and other organs, the more severe the results can be.

Treatment for Wilson's Disease includes chelating agents, which encourage the release of stored copper into your organs into your bloodstream. There it can be filtered, processed, and excreted by your kidneys and urinary system. In severe or extreme cases, medication may not be enough, and a liver transplant may be required.

*Alcohol-Related Liver Disease*

Probably the most widely known cause of liver disease is alcohol abuse.

Women are more likely to develop alcohol-related liver disease, but nearly all heavy drinkers will develop fatty liver disease. Other forms of alcohol-related liver disease are cirrhosis and alcoholic hepatitis, but in all cases, alcohol consumption is the trigger of the disease.

If alcoholic liver disease is caught early, the damage to the liver can be reversed, provided the person stops drinking. Later stage treatments will also all require that you quit drinking completely.

Alcohol is a toxin. In moderate amounts, our livers can process it and filter it, and it does not do too much damage. But when you drink excessively, your liver cannot cope, and the toxins buildup and damage your liver. The longer you continue to drink, the more damage you will do.

If your liver is irreparably damaged by alcohol abuse, a liver transplant would be the only option for a cure. Still, in many countries, a liver transplant will only be considered if you have been alcohol-free for six months to a year.

*Cirrhosis*

Cirrhosis is a liver condition caused by long term scarring on the organ. It can be triggered by any one of the other conditions mentioned here, and it is a secondary condition. Every time your liver is injured, whether by disease or by alcohol abuse, scar tissue forms when it tries to repair itself. Over time, this scar tissue builds up, preventing the liver from working properly.

There are many causes of cirrhosis, but the top three are alcohol abuse, being overweight (which can cause conditions like fatty liver), and viral hepatitis.

The longer cirrhosis goes untreated or undiagnosed, the more serious it becomes. The condition can be fatal if appropriate action is not taken. Cirrhosis can also trigger secondary conditions of its own, including high blood pressure, bleeding, bone conditions, toxin buildup, and liver cancer.

To diagnose cirrhosis, your doctor may use a combination of imaging tests like MRIs and CT scans, blood tests, and possibly a liver biopsy.

Because cirrhosis is a secondary condition caused by something else, cirrhosis treatment is always related to the underlying cause. Your doctor will recommend lifestyle changes like avoiding alcohol and changing your diet, losing weight, and medication to treat diseases like hepatitis. If you have developed related conditions like high blood pressure, fluid buildup, or infections as a result of having cirrhosis, your doctor will treat those too.

*Liver Cancer*

Liver cancer can start in the liver (primary liver cancer) or spread there from somewhere else (secondary liver cancer.) Cancer causes the cells of the liver to stop behaving normally, and mutations start to occur. These mutations result in tumors, which in the case of liver cancer, we call malignant tumors.

The most common (although not only) type of liver cancer is cancer that affects the hepatocytes, which are the cells that make up most of your liver.

It is much rarer to get a primary form of liver cancer. In most cases, liver cancer is secondary and spreads or metastasizes to your liver from somewhere else in your body. When primary liver cancer does occur, it is usually the result of some other form of liver condition, alcohol abuse, smoking, diabetes, using certain kinds of birth control, and other lifestyle factors.

Some people will get liver cancer even though they take good care of themselves. In most cases, however, making healthier choices in your lifestyle, being on the lookout for liver disease symptoms, and taking steps to treat liver conditions if you are diagnosed with one, will lower your risk.

Symptoms of liver cancer depend on the type of cancer you have. They may include common liver disease symptoms, like abdominal pain, nausea, vomiting, loss of appetite, and fatigue. You may also have digestive issues like diarrhea or constipation.

In less common types of liver cancer like hepatic encephalopathy, stranger symptoms like changes in the way your breath smells, and personality changes may also be experienced.

As with any cancer, the sooner liver cancer is diagnosed, and treatment begins, the better your long-term prognosis will be. If you have any strange symptoms, and particularly if you have another liver condition, seek expert medical care as soon as possible. Your doctor will want to run many tests, ranging from blood tests to imaging and scans, possibly a biopsy and others. It can be a long and scary process, but the sooner you start, the better your outcomes will likely be.

Once you have been diagnosed with liver cancer, your doctor will do what is known as "staging," which is assessing the nature and spread of your cancer. They will assign it a stage between 0 (less severe) and D (more severe), which determines the severity. This will be a factor in determining the type of treatment you get.

There are various treatments for liver cancer, including radiation, chemotherapy, surgery, and others. Many patients will have a combination of treatments. Even after cancer is "cured," your doctor will want to monitor you regularly because liver cancer (like many others) can recur.

*Fatty Liver Disease*

Fatty liver disease refers to any condition where there is more than 5% fat built up in the liver. When this buildup is caused by alcohol abuse, it is the first stage of what is known as ARLD or Alcohol-Related Liver Disease.

Fatty liver disease does not usually have any noticeable symptoms. When it is caused by alcohol, quitting drinking is the only treatment necessary to reverse the damage. In fact, if you stop drinking for as little as two weeks during the early stages of ARLD, your liver will be able to repair itself, and that should solve the problem.

It's important to note that fatty liver disease, in general, is related to being overweight or obese. So if you drink more than you should and are carrying a few extra pounds, you have a higher risk of developing this condition.

### *Non-Alcoholic Fatty Liver Disease*

Non-alcoholic fatty liver disease or NAFLD is a type of fatty liver disease that is not related to alcohol. In fact, it can even affect children. There is also another type of non-alcohol related fatty liver disease, known as NASH, or Non-Alcoholic Steatohepatitis. Of the two, NASH is much more severe and significantly increases patients' risk of developing liver cancer.

"Normal" fatty liver generally does not have too many symptoms and is mostly a benign condition. However, people who have NASH tend to have more symptoms, often develop secondary conditions like cirrhosis, and have long-term damage as a result.

In both NAFLD and NASH, as with alcohol-related fatty liver disease, the buildup of fat in the liver makes the liver more "fragile" and vulnerable to damage. The disease itself is not a problem, but if you have any other liver conditions, such as hepatitis, you could experience profoundly serious complications.

There are no specific treatments for NAFLD and NASH, but since they are far more prevalent in people who are overweight or obese, your doctor will almost certainly prescribe lifestyle changes, including a healthier diet and more exercise.

Your doctor will also want to monitor your liver and be on a special alert for secondary conditions that you may develop over time.

## Drug-Related Liver Disease

While this list of conditions is not exhaustive, and many other, rarer conditions could affect your liver, the last of the more common problems we are going to cover is drug-related liver disease.

As we have already established, your liver is a filter for most things you eat and put into your body. That includes alcohol and drugs, whether legal or otherwise.

Some people who develop drug-related liver disease have been prescribed a medication where there is potential for liver damage. Still, there tend to be more cases with people who use illicit drugs.

When you are taking prescription medication where there is a risk of liver damage, your doctor will carefully monitor it, so it is much less likely to happen. If it does, it will be caught quickly. When you are taking recreational, illegal drugs, no one monitors how your body reacts. Over time, that can result in serious problems.

There are various kinds of drug-related liver disease you might experience, such as drug-induced hepatitis or drug-induced cholestasis. In all of these kinds of disease, however, the drugs themselves trigger the condition, affecting your liver function and leading to long-term scarring and other potential problems.

Symptoms of drug-related liver disease will mirror the non-drug-related disease's signs, with some of the most common being fatigue, jaundice, abdominal pain and swelling, or bloating.

If you are taking drugs, prescription or otherwise, and notice any signs and symptoms of liver disease, it is important that you consult your doctor as soon as possible to confirm or rule out liver disease caused by the drugs. As with most types of liver disease with lifestyle or environmental factors, one of the most important things is to remove the trigger or cause. Which may mean changing prescription medication or avoiding recreational drug use.

Not all liver diseases caused by drug use can be reversed by removing the trigger. Still, it will always be a factor in the treatment plan recommended by your doctor.

## The Golden Rules of Liver Disease

Your liver is a complex, vital biological "machine" that your body needs to perform hundreds of functions in one way or another. As with most conditions, the earlier you catch and start to treat any kind of liver disease, the better your outcomes will be long term.

Learn to listen to your body and notice symptoms that might be a cause for concern. Then, consult a doctor as soon as possible when you feel something is off.

Never ignore symptoms like abdominal pain, jaundice, bloating or swelling, and gastrointestinal problems that do not go away within a few days.

Liver diseases often start very mild and get worse over time. They also tend to trigger secondary conditions as they progress, which makes treating them later significantly more complicated.

It is always worrisome to have unexplained medical symptoms. The temptation is always to pretend they are not there, but that will not have the desired effect.

Most liver conditions can be treated and managed. You can also make easy, natural changes to your lifestyle to stop them from worsening, or in many cases, reverse some or all of the damage. So be brave, tackle the problem head-on, and you will have a better result.

> He who has health has hope; and he who has hope has everything.

*Arabic Proverb*

# 3

# IMPROVING LIVER HEALTH

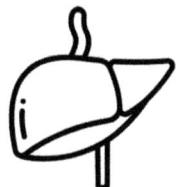

So far, the information in this book has been more of an introduction to the general concepts of liver health, and what might be affecting your liver's function. It is time to get down to the meat and potatoes of the book, though.

If you don't suffer from a liver-related disease, this chapter will show you how to take proactive and preemptive measures to avoid it. If you do have a liver condition, it will show you how to support whatever medical advice you have been given.

After all, as the 19th century, American philosopher William James said: *"Is life worth living? It depends on the liver."*

He might have been making a clever play on words. Still, your liver really does play a major role in every aspect of your health, and therefore your life. There isn't a single person who won't find some benefit in having a healthier liver.

Simple Changes, Big Results

Reading about how liver health can be life-changing might make you worry that it will be complicated or expensive to improve yours. Or that you will need to buy all sorts of expensive pills, potions, and supplements.

The good news is that this is not the case. In fact, the opposite is true.

The keys to improving the health and functioning of one of the most complex and miraculous organs in your body is simple. It won't require much if any investment and can be made in easy stages, so you don't have to make big, drastic changes all at once.

We recommend making one or two small changes every week, giving yourself time to adjust, and then moving on to the next step. After all, building better habits is all about repetition. You are far more likely to stick to the changes you make if you continue to progress with your goals slowly over some time.

We also recommend discussing any major changes you plan to make to your lifestyle with your doctor. Particularly if you have an existing condition, or you are going through a lifestyle change. This may include trying to get pregnant, being pregnant, nursing, starting or going through menopause, and more. All of these things can have an effect on your body's needs and capabilities, and should always be factored in.

Most of the changes we recommend in this chapter are based on two major areas of your health and lifestyle: nutrition and exercise. Let's get to it!

Nutrition and Your Liver

Aside from the specific benefit to your liver health, it is useful to think of the food you eat as fuel for the complex machine that is your body. The higher the quality of the fuel and the more efficiently it gets the job done, the better the machine works.

This is true for every system in your body, but because it is involved in digesting or processing that "fuel," even more so for your liver.

**Nutrition Basics**

Most people do not put too much thought into what they eat. Those that do are often taken in by fads and trends that do not necessarily have any noticeable benefit. So, we thought we would start with the very basics of nutrition, so you can start to understand the science of food, and what it does for and to your body. Here is what you need to know in broad strokes.

*Macronutrients*

Macronutrients are the nutrients that you need in larger amounts every single day.

There are three major types of macronutrients: carbohydrates, proteins, and fats. We need all three of those to be healthy, but the ratios and quality of the foods we get them from go a long way to determining how well we can process and use them.

**Carbohydrates** are "fast fuel" for your body. They are the first thing your body uses as energy for the cells and systems that make up your body.

There are two main types of carbohydrates: *simple carbohydrates* that are usually refined and processed quickly, causing a sharp spike in blood sugars and *complex carbohydrates*, which take longer to process, and typically include things like fiber, which are also important to overall health.

Most modern nutritional wisdom recommends choosing complex carbs over simple ones. So, choose whole grains, starchy vegetables, and whole fruits rather than things like white bread and rice, refined sugar, and fruit juice. These offer extraordinarily little nutritional value and can actually trigger or exacerbate inflammatory conditions and other diet-related problems.

Most healthy people need to get between 45 and 65% of their daily nutrients from carbohydrates. However, it is recommended that most of those are complex carbs.

**Protein** is the next essential macronutrient your body needs to function at its peak. High-quality proteins like meats, fish, poultry, eggs, vegetables, dairy products, and legumes all contain amino acids. Your body needs this to build muscle, and carry out repairs on damaged tissue. This is particularly important for your liver since it is always working to keep itself in good condition!

Your body actually manufactures eleven amino acids of its own. Still, there are nine that it cannot make, which you have to get from your daily diet to stay in the best possible health.

Your body can also do some other impressive stuff with protein, including converting it into energy through a process called gluconeogenesis, so if you do not get enough energy from carbohydrates, you have a backup plan!

Proteins are divided into complete proteins (usually from animal sources) and incomplete proteins (usually from plant sources.) While that doesn't mean you can't get enough protein on a plant-based diet, it does mean that you need to be even more careful to get all the amino acids you need to stay healthy if you do.

Most dietary authorities now recommend that you get between 10 and 30% of your daily calories from protein-based foods.

**Fats** have a bad reputation, but they are actually essential for many processes in our bodies, including important things like brain function. Stored fat can be used as energy when needed, and a little fat on our bodies is important for insulation. We also need fat for many cell functions, and to protect our organs.

However, when it comes to fat, it is very much a quality over quantity situation!

High-quality unsaturated fats, usually from plant-based sources, and typically liquid even when refrigerated, are the fat of choice for a healthy diet. Choose nuts, avocados, olive oil, and seed oils. Essential fats are also present in a few animal sources, like Omega 3 enriched eggs and fatty seafood.

Saturated fats, however, are the kind we need to be incredibly careful around. Animal fats like bacon grease, butter, visible fat on meats, and similar are generally solid at room temperature, and it is these fats that are typically associated with clogging arteries and other undesirable effects.

Whenever you can, choose healthy fats over unhealthy, and avoid highly processed foods that contain trans fats.

It may be surprising, but dieticians usually recommend that you get between 20 and 35% of your daily calories from fats – but no more than 10% of those from saturated fats. Remember, however, that all fats are high calorie. So if you want to lose weight, you may need to reduce your overall calories, including those from fat, while you work to reduce that number!

That might sound like a lot of "food math," but when you get used to balancing your meals, making healthy choices in macronutrients becomes a lot easier. As a general rule of thumb, the less processed your foods are, the better they will be for you, and home-cooked is always better than bought because you can control what you put in every dish.

*Micronutrients*

If macronutrients are like the broad strokes of a healthy diet, then micronutrients can be seen as the details.

Micronutrients are things like vitamins and minerals that perform specific functions in your body. We all need these nutrients to keep everything running smoothly. When you do not get enough of a particular type of micronutrient, you will develop a deficiency. When that happens, you can incur some unpleasant and potentially dangerous conditions. Of course, you need many micronutrients, but here are some of the more important ones you need to pay attention to.

**Iron** is an essential trace element that your body needs to transport oxygen around your body, and for many other functions. Unless you have a condition like hemochromatosis, you need to make sure that you eat enough iron-rich foods to keep your blood iron levels within healthy ranges for your age, gender, and weight.

When you do not get enough iron, you can develop a condition called anemia, which can be dangerous or life-threatening.

We get iron from animal-based sources like red meat, as well as plant-based sources like leafy greens and beans, tofu and fortified grain products. However, it is important to note that there is a difference between animal-based or haem iron and non-haem iron from plant sources. Research shows that the former is processed more easily and is therefore, more "bioavailable." This means that people who avoid animal products should pay close attention to their iron levels and supplement when necessary.

It is also worth noting that eating iron-rich foods with foods or drinks containing vitamin C will help promote absorption.

**Vitamin A**, also known as retinol, is another especially important micronutrient. It supports eyesight, as well as immune function, growth, reproductive function, and cell division. People who have a vitamin A deficiency are more likely to have problems like night blindness and are more likely to be sickly.

We get vitamin A from a wide variety of foods, including dark leafy greens, foods that contain beta carotene like carrots, liver, and dairy products. There are also many supplements that contain vitamin A, however, unless you are not getting enough vitamin A from the food you eat, they are not necessary to overall health.

Too much vitamin A can also cause problems of its own, including liver damage over the long term. So, unless your doctor recommends a supplement, be cautious about adding any to your diet.

**Vitamin D**, also known as the sunshine vitamin, is one that we tend to get from exposure to sunlight. Still, it is also available from a limited number of foods, like fatty fish, including salmon and herring, cod liver oil, canned tuna, along with mushrooms and egg yolks.

However, it's important to note that as many as 50% of the world's population do not get enough vitamin D from food or the sun. This makes it one of the micronutrients where many of us can benefit from a supplement.

Signs that you might not be getting enough vitamin D include problems with bone density, muscle and nerve conditions, and a weak immune system.

If you live in a part of the world where there is limited sunlight, it can be recommended to speak to your doctor about taking a vitamin D supplement as part of your daily routine.

**Iodine** is another micronutrient that we need in order to be as healthy as possible. Low iodine levels can lead to potentially serious problems like thyroid problems, reproductive problems, brain function issues, and trouble healing from injuries.

Iodine is present in fish and seafood, dairy products, and some fruits and vegetables. It's also been added to salt in many countries (you will see the term "iodized" on the label!). However, you will want to avoid excess salt intake because it can lead to other problems like hypertension.

As many as 1.8 billion people worldwide are estimated to have an iodine deficiency, mainly because it is extremely hard to get enough from diet alone.

If you are worried that you are not getting enough iodine in your diet, it is a good idea to speak to your doctor about a supplement that might make up the difference. This is especially important if you are pregnant or planning to get pregnant because iodine is particularly important to fetal brain development!

**Folate** is another vital trace element that we need to get from our diet.

The micronutrient is necessary to make DNA and to help your cells to divide. So, it is literally essential to your health on a cellular level. Folate is also great for pregnant women as it reduces the risk of neural tube defects in their babies.

Folate is present in many different kinds of foods, including beef liver, green and dark green vegetables, including asparagus, brussels sprouts, and spinach, in fruits and fruit juices (especially oranges and orange juice) and in beans and legumes. Many foods are also "enriched" with folate or folic acid, which means it is added to the food during the manufacturing process, like fortified bread products.

Women of childbearing age, in particular, might want to consider a folic acid supplement. If you are pregnant, remember to take prenatal vitamins – it is crucial for your baby's development!

**Zinc** is the last micronutrient we are going to look at in detail. This micronutrient is essential for immune function, making DNA, healing wounds, and manufacturing the amino acids that our bodies make themselves.

The best source for zinc is oysters, but you can also get this micronutrient from red meat, poultry, and other types of seafood. It is also in beans, nuts, seeds, dairy products, and whole grains.

Most healthy people will get enough zinc from their diet because we only need a little to keep everything working properly. However, if you have a digestive condition like Crohn's, are vegetarian, an alcoholic, or have sickle cell disease, you may need a supplement.

Of course, there are many other vitamins, minerals, and trace elements we need to maintain optimal health. Still, most are needed in much smaller doses, and will easily be absorbed from most diets.

It is always recommended to follow a healthy diet, "eat the rainbow," and try not to completely eliminate any food groups without talking to your doctor.

*Antioxidants*

So far, we have mainly been discussing the nutrients that we need for specific functions. Antioxidants are a little different, because instead of using them to do something specific, they are used to protect and repair all of our cells.

Just by being alive, our cells are constantly being bombarded by potentially damaging threats. Most of these threats are due to what are called "free radicals," which are unstable molecules that are all around us all the time.

As we interact with free radicals, our cells become damaged, which leaves us vulnerable to some unpleasant side effects. These could range from deficiencies to bacteria and viruses and even cancer. While our body works to repair that damage, antioxidants help our cells to resist damage. Since prevention is always better than cure, that is an especially important function!

Antioxidants effectively neutralize free radicals, making it safer for us to interact with the world in our daily lives.

*Where Do We Get Antioxidants?*

Antioxidants include vitamins like vitamins C and E, flavonoids, phenols, tannins, and lignans. We get them mainly from the food we eat, and primarily from plant-based foods.

The good news is that there are a wide range of antioxidant sources, from spices to cocoa, to vegetables and fruit, nuts, seeds, and grains. So, there is guaranteed to be at least a few foods you love that contain a lot of antioxidants.

*How to Make Sure You Get Enough Antioxidants.*

When it comes to antioxidants, there really is no "too much of a good thing." More is better, and the easiest way to make sure you are getting enough is to stick to the old wisdom of "eating the rainbow."

Choose a variety of fruits, vegetables, berries, nuts, and grains, and try to eat them raw whenever possible. Add nuts and sunflower seeds to your diet, choose wholegrain products, and opt for smoothies and freshly squeezed juices whenever you can.

The more natural, whole, colorful, plant-based foods you can add to your diet, the more antioxidants you will be giving your body to fight off free radicals. It is food, but also preventative medicine!

*Phytochemicals*

The last section in our lesson on nutrition for better liver health is phytochemicals. These food sourced chemicals are actually one of the newer discoveries in the world of nutrition and health, and as such, there is still a lot of in-depth studies happening.

*What Are Phytochemicals?*

The word *"Phyto"* means plant in ancient Greek. In other words, phytochemicals are chemicals that come from plants. They are the chemicals that give plants their scent, taste, and color, but they also have health benefits when we eat them.

Phytochemicals give carrots their color and chili peppers their sting. Still, they are found throughout plants, in all parts of fruits, vegetables, nuts, seeds, and legumes, including and sometimes especially in the rind or peel.

*What Do Phytochemicals DO?*

Science is still learning about phytochemicals. With over 5,000 (and counting) discovered so far, it is almost impossible to say what all of them do, and what the benefits are to our bodies. However, thanks to smart people around the world, there are many that we have cataloged, and these are some of the benefits you get from phytochemicals you eat:

- Carotenoids are the chemicals that give the color to orange, red, yellow, and green foods. They are particularly bioavailable when cooked, especially in tomatoes, carrots, broccoli, and squash. They have been shown to help reduce

instances of cancer, heart disease, and boost the immune system.
- Flavonoids, which are the chemicals that give fruits, berries, and even coffee their flavor and aroma. They are believed to fight tumor growth and prevent or limit inflammation.
- Red wine lovers will be happy to learn about the phytochemical, resveratrol. It can be found in red wine, grapes, peanuts, and dark chocolate, and it has been linked to a longer lifespan... Enjoy in moderation!
- Anthocyanins, which we also get from berries and red wine, have been shown to lower blood pressure.
- Flavanols and proanthocyanins, which are available from cocoa, apples, grapes and red wine, help reduce blood pressure and preserve the lining of the arteries.
- Sulfides and thiols, which give vegetables like olives, leeks, scallions, onions, and garlic their signature pungency, have been linked to lower LDL or "bad" cholesterol.
- Terpenes, in citrus fruit and cherries, help to fight cancer cell growth and can help to protect against viruses.
- Lutein and zeaxanthin, which we find in dark leafy greens, have been linked to better visual health.

There are thousands of other phytochemicals out there, all from different sources, and all with various benefits. Science is still discovering what these remarkable natural compounds can do for us. Since studying anything related to health involved long-term real-life studies and lab-based research, it will be a while before we have the whole picture.

There is one fact that most studies have discovered and confirmed, though – the benefits we get from phytochemicals are exclusively related to a healthy diet. You cannot cheat by eating badly and then taking a pill.

### How to Get More Phytochemicals in Your Diet.

While we do not know what all the phytochemicals are or what they do, we know that they have significant health benefits and come from brightly colored, highly flavored, scented plant-based foods.

So, the best way to get more of the good stuff these compounds offer in your life is to eat between five and nine servings of fruits and vegetables every day, and to mix it up as much as you can. If you do not love one (kale, we are looking at you!), try another, like asparagus or broccoli.

More than ever, it is clear that eating more plant-derived foods is critical to our overall health, and of course, since it has a finger in nearly every biological pie, to your liver health in particular.

## The Healthy Liver Diet

Now that we know the general basics of good nutrition, it's time to get down to specifics you can target to improve liver function and health.

### Choose Whole Foods

The first thing you should be doing is choosing whole foods wherever possible. Processed foods, by definition, contain a lot of additives, chemicals, and other stuff. Since your liver is the organ that has to process all that "stuff" out of your system, it's the one that has to work harder when you make bad choices.

There are some benefits to organic foods, but remember that organic does not mean pesticide-free – it is just a different kind of pesticide! Make sure you also wash and prepare foods carefully, because all those chemicals (even the organic ones) can take a toll on your liver as well!

Fresh fruits and vegetables, leafy greens, legumes, nuts and seeds, and some whole grains should make up the bulk of your diet and foundation. Lean meats, proteins, and some healthy oils will be situated at the top of the "pyramid."

*Eat More Fiber*

Your liver is part of the digestive tract, so another big part of its function is making sure that waste makes it out of your body. Fiber is "natures broom", helping to bulk up that waste material and keep things moving.

Fiber is abundantly present in fruits, vegetables, and whole grains. So, making smart food choices is the first step in getting things moving. If all else fails, your doctor may recommend adding a fiber supplement like psyllium, which is present in many drinks and preparations. It does not have much of a nutritional impact aside from improving your bowel function.

*Add Garlic to Your Diet*

Sure... It's not great for romance (unless you are romancing a fellow garlic lover!), but it is excellent for your liver!

Garlic contains a lot of selenium, which is a mineral that helps to detoxify your liver. It helps to "activate" liver enzymes, which makes it easier for your liver to do its job.

*Vitamin C*

Vitamin C, from citrus fruits like oranges, grapefruit, and lemons, helps to promote the production of liver enzymes and improves the detoxifying abilities of your liver. Just a little bit of vitamin C from citrus or other sources like apples, tomatoes, and sweet peppers can boost your liver's cleansing abilities.

*Turmeric*

It is well known that many spices are "superfoods", but few have shown themselves to be as effective as turmeric. This golden yellow spice, popular in Indian and other cuisines, does a whole lot of particularly essential things for your liver!

It supports the enzymes that flush out toxins and contains antioxidants that repair free radical damage to liver cells. It helps the liver to detox from metals that we get from our diet. Last, but certainly not least, this golden super spice also helps to increase bile production.

*Walnuts*

All nuts are good for us, but Walnuts are particularly important for liver health because they contain glutathione and omega 3 fatty acids. These help cleanse the liver and, more importantly, the amino acid arginine, which helps the liver process and eliminate ammonia.

### Apples

Apples not only contain vitamin C, which is good for your liver, but they also contain pectin, which supports cleansing and eliminating toxins from the liver. Pectin is also available from pears, guavas, quince, plums, and gooseberries. So a fruit salad is a great way to support your liver health, and it's tasty too!

### Avocados

You have probably heard of the benefits of the fatty acids in avocados, but how about their ability to assist in the production of glutathione, which helps the liver expel toxins? Add their natural ability to help "clean" your arteries for better blood flow to your liver and everything else, and this is one superfood you need on your liver health menu!

### Green Tea

Green tea contains a phytochemical known as catechins, which are known to improve liver function. As always though, choose the real thing over extracts and derivatives, because some of those can do more harm than good.

### Milk Thistle

Milk thistle, also referred to as Silybum Marianum, is a plant that is well known to support liver function. The primary function it performs is to prevent toxins from attaching themselves to liver cells, which makes it easier for your liver to expel them from your body. It has also been shown to reduce inflammation and help to prevent or treat liver diseases and disorders.

Since many milk thistle preparations are sold as herbal medication, and they can vary in safety and efficacy, it's a good idea to discuss taking milk thistle with your doctor. Ask them to recommend a product that is safe and effective.

*Dandelion Greens*

Nope, they aren't just a weed. Dandelion greens might be something you always pulled out of your lawn, but they are actually proven to pack some impressive health benefits as well. Particularly for your liver.

Dandelion greens are well known to support liver and kidney function. They are extremely easy to incorporate into your diet. Simply add some to your next salad for a bitter crunch and some added liver love.

Drinks for Liver Health

While we may have said that red wine has some health benefits (in moderation) when it comes to your liver, it is best to keep it simple and alcohol-free! Liver friendly drinks are simple and help dilute and flush out toxins, so your liver does not have to work so hard.

Choose water, lemon water, green tea, and freshly made juices and smoothies with any of the foods we mentioned above to give your liver a liquid boost.

Avoid drinks with added sugar, commercial juices, which have extraordinarily little nutritional value and no fiber and limit your alcohol intake whenever possible.

Body and Soul

Good health and good liver health may be built on what you put into your body, but it is supported by what you **DO** with your body.

If food is the fuel that drives your body's engine, then your lifestyle is the preventative maintenance that keeps it in tip-top condition. There are some remarkably simple, fundamental lifestyle choices that help you maintain good health, and in turn, support good liver health.

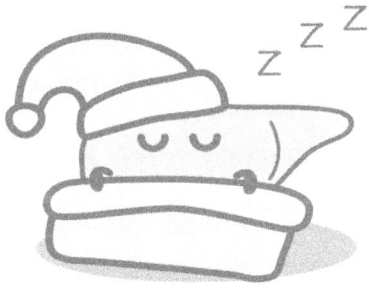

*Sleep*

Never underestimate the power of sleep.

Research paper after research paper has shown that it is crucial in keeping your body weight down, helping to prevent and treat certain diseases, and critical to give your body time to heal and repair itself.

Sleep is important for physical health, but also for cognitive function. We all know how much "less" we feel when we are sleep deprived!

Sleep has even been shown to be linked to a longer lifespan. So, make time to sleep. Make your bedroom a restful, peaceful place where you can truly relax. Turn off the devices. Meditate, take time to relax, and aim for at least seven to eight hours per night.

If you do find yourself dealing with sleep debt or are feeling particularly tired, listen to your body. A short power nap can improve your mood and your health!

*Exercise*

If you thought exercise was just about having a hard body, think again.

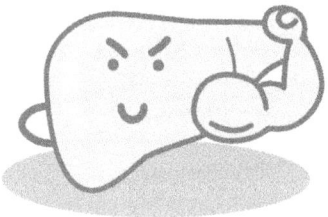

Exercise has so many health benefits, from improving mental health to helping your digestive system do its job.

You do not have to take up marathon running either, a brisk walk in the park, a bike ride with your kids, or a sweaty dance session in your living room all count. The more you move your body, the better it is for your overall health and your liver!

*De-Stress*

Stress is known as the silent killer.

It has been linked to heart disease, cancer, and other serious conditions. It changes the way we eat, sleep, and interact with one another. It can suck the joy out of life, so we are not motivated to take care of ourselves.

If you find yourself self-medicating your stress or comfort eating things you know are not good for you, you need to take steps to manage your stress levels.

There are things you can change when it comes to your life's stress levels, like distancing yourself from toxic people, but there will always be some stressful situations. Learn skills that help you manage stress. Learn to say no. Learn to take time for yourself. Learn to sometimes just do nothing but focus your mind on yourself.

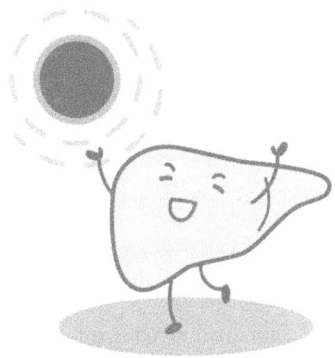

### Things to Avoid

Just like there are things you need to seek out to improve your liver health, there are many things you should avoid to preserve it. These are some of the most important.

#### *Smoking and Alcohol*

There may be some minor benefits to some types of alcohol in moderation. But there are really no benefits to smoking at all.

Cigarette smoke has been proven to negatively impact everything from brain function and fertility, to bone density and eyesight. It is bad for your teeth, terrible for your lungs, costs a small fortune, and makes you smell like an ashtray.

Because it also funnels dozens of highly toxic, potentially lethal chemicals into your body, your liver also has to work extra hard to remove those poisons from your system. If you still smoke, it is time to stop. Your whole body, including your liver, will thank you!

Where alcohol is concerned, it is important to remember the word "moderation." A glass of wine, or even two, will not destroy your liver. However, consistent consumption will have negative effects on your overall health and especially that of your liver.

#### *Too Much Fat*

As we discussed, we need some fats to live a healthy life. Most of these are vegetable-based fats, and most are unprocessed.

If you are overeating unhealthy fat from animal sources, or deep-fried foods with very little nutritional value and a whole lot of grease, or highly processed foods with hydrogenated and trans fats, then you are getting the wrong kind of fat.

Start a food diary and take note of what you are eating every day. Most of your foods should be unprocessed and home-cooked, and you should be trimming off visible fat on meats and other proteins. Deep-fried foods should be an occasional treat.

Too much fat can lead to weight gain, and that can lead to fatty liver disease, which is the starting point of many more severe liver conditions. Take steps now to make better choices, and you will benefit later on.

*Pesticides*

Pesticides, no matter which kind they are, are not good for us. They are made to kill bugs, which makes it clear that we are not going to get any benefit from them.

Make sure that you wash fruits and vegetables very carefully, and when there is any doubt, peeling the skin off before preparing them is a good idea.

Remember that this applies to organic and non-organic produce too. Organic does not mean pesticide-free – it is simply different pesticides, so you still need to wash or peel those fruits and vegetables.

If you have the space and the time, it is never a bad idea to grow some of your own produce as well. Just like a home-cooked meal, there is nothing like knowing exactly what went into growing your produce!

. . .

*Drugs*

Whether it is a prescription from your doctor, or recreational drugs on the weekend, if you are taking it, your liver is processing it. Sometimes, that can be bad news for your liver.

If you have been prescribed medication by your doctor, always ask about possible side effects, and only take medication according to your doctor's instructions.

If you notice any signs of liver trouble while you are taking medication, speak to your doctor as soon as possible. Symptoms like abdominal pain, jaundice, and nausea can all be early signs of drug-related liver injury or disease.

Mental Health Issues

A study in Edinburgh recently discovered a link between poor mental health, including stress, anxiety and depression, and potential damage to your liver. The study did not conclude whether the mental health conditions themselves caused the liver problems or whether secondary symptoms of those conditions like obesity, alcohol and drug abuse, and increased stress hormones were to blame.

But the simple fact is that your mental health has a profound impact on everything in your body, including your liver.

Review Prescriptions

Food and nutrition are a huge part of improving liver health. Still, if you are on prescription medications, they may also be affecting your liver function.

It is good to review your prescription medications with your doctor if you notice that you are experiencing signs of trouble with your liver (or anything else.) Prescription medications can be lifesaving, but they can also have significant side effects.

Medications and medical science changes over time, as does your health. So, there may be new treatments that are better suited to whatever condition you have, which have less impact on other things in your body.

You should never stop taking prescription medication without the approval and supervision of your doctor. Still, if you are concerned, a conversation about your options is an excellent place to start.

Build Liver Detox into Your Life

Generally, doctors do not recommend detoxing for the sake of detox. However, when it comes to your liver, it is a critical part of maintaining and improving liver health. This will boost your energy, improve your metabolism, and even improve the appearance of your hair, skin, and waistline. When your liver is working at its peak, it will do everything better and more efficiently, and that will show in every area of your life.

Life gets busy. Maybe you are eating more take-out pizza than you should because you are working late. Perhaps you have been having a few too many after-work cocktails. Or maybe you are just noticing that you are feeling more tired than usual. If you are, here are 8 simple steps you can take right now to do your own liver detox and get things back on track.

For the next week, do these simple things:

1. Switch all your usual drinks for water or green tea.

2. Cut out all processed foods, whether that is take out or commercially prepared sauces and snacks.

3. Include 7 to 9 servings of fruit and vegetables per day.

4. Limit protein intake to lean meat, poultry, and fish, eggs, or legumes and vegetables.

5. Ban all processed sugar and flour. Choose only whole grain products.

6. Make sure that you eat three balanced meals every day and two healthy snacks.

7. Get enough sleep.

8. Get 30 minutes of low impact exercise every second day.

These straightforward steps are all you need to begin improving your liver health. Give it time to heal from the damage of everyday life, and get yourself feeling better.

You do not need any special pills or supplements, and it does not cost a lot of money or take a lot of time. Treating your liver right is as simple as living a healthier lifestyle. Because your liver can repair and regenerate itself, even if you have not been doing everything right, you can start today.

Weight Loss and Liver Health

While we all know the link between alcohol, smoking, drugs, and liver damage, the truth is that many liver disease cases are not related to any of those things. There is a large body of evidence that shows that being overweight or obese is one of the leading causes of liver disease.

That means that losing weight is one of the best ways to improve your liver health and function.

If you are carrying extra weight, especially in your abdomen, there is a good chance you are at risk of fatty liver disease or might already have the early stages of the condition.

Speak to your doctor to determine what a healthy weight goal is, and use the tips and recipes in this book, combined with moderate exercise and your doctor's advice to lose weight slowly and sustainably.

We are all for positive body image at any weight. Still, if you are putting your liver at risk by carrying extra pounds, it might be time to make some small changes to reap significant health benefits.

### You are in the Driver's Seat

We hope that this chapter helped show you how much control you actually have over your liver health – and your health in general.

The simplest things, like choosing the right foods and making smart lifestyle choices, can all have a profound impact on everything in our bodies, including our liver health. When we take good care of our bodies, our bodies will take care of us.

Good health is a self-fulfilling prophecy in that way. The more we make better choices, the more benefits we will see, and the more benefits we see, the more we will want to make smarter choices.

It all starts with a choice, though. Choose to make small changes that have a big impact, and you will start to see big changes in your health and wellbeing.

But what about the damage that you might have already done? Many people feel that it is too late to make smart choices because they have already made too many bad ones. We want you to know that it's never too late to change, and that brings us to the next chapter in this book: how to start undoing some of the bad choices you might have made, by detoxing your liver and your life.

> You can't control what goes on outside, but you CAN control what goes on inside.

*Unknown*

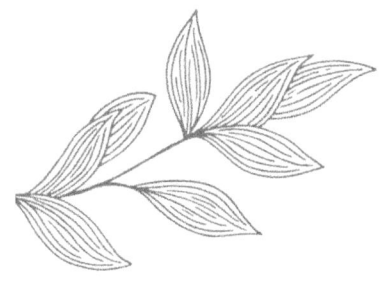

# Detox & Cleanse

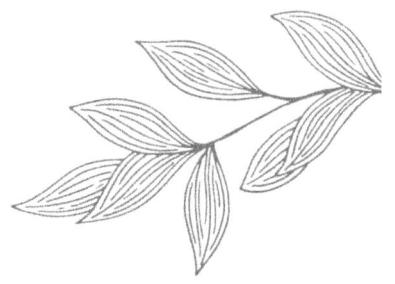

## DETOX & CLEANSE

There are two approaches to health and wellness.

The first focuses on the cosmetic, clear skin, shiny hair, or a slimmer waistline.

The second focuses on creating better habits, so you can get sustained and sustainable health benefits for the rest of your life.

While the first approach initially feels the most appealing and is the most popular advertising strategy, it is not based on anything real. It is like the crash diets of health. As soon as you stop doing the (usually impossible to maintain) things they recommend, everything goes back to what it was before. Or, in the case of most crash diets, it gets even worse.

That is why we are not focused on quick fixes, gimmicks, or cosmetic change.

We're not going to even consider so-called "cleanses" that cut your calories so much that they put you into starvation mode and do more harm than good, and we're not going to sell you a miracle potion.

In this book, we are only looking at genuine, long term changes that you can make a part of your lifestyle, to get better liver health, and experience the health benefits that come along with that.

As the famous nutritionist Fiona Tuck says, "The body is naturally designed to be able to clear waste materials such as toxins, chemicals and old hormones in order to prevent an accumulation of potentially toxic and harmful byproducts from building up in our systems."

Your body already knows how to do what needs to be done. So, we are going to teach you how to get out of its way, so it can get the job done. As Hippocrates said, "Let food be thy medicine, and medicine be thy food." So, let us learn how to eat the right foods to promote healing, let our livers do the miraculous job they were created to do, and start living a healthier, more energetic, more enjoyable life.

But because we need to make sure you stick to your new, healthier lifestyle, let us also make sure they are filling, delicious, and satisfying. All recipes are designed for one person but can easily be adjusted if you are feeding more people.

**\*A special note about the recipes:** Some of the dishes include meat. Alternatively, these can be made as vegetarian options. Simply don't add the meat or replace it with an extra serving of your favorite vegetable or meat replacement. Popular replacement options include tofu, tempeh, jackfruit, mushrooms, lentils, beans, and legumes.

Some recipes will also include honey to sweeten a dish. Please use this in moderation. Honey has been linked to improved heart health, blood antioxidant status, and wound healing. Still, it does contain plenty of sugar and calories. Consuming too much will have adverse effects.

In general, the recipes can be modified to your liking depending on what diet you follow (vegetarian or vegan).

# BREAKFAST

They say it is the most important meal of the day, and when it comes to energy, weight loss, detoxing, and metabolism, they are not lying!

We have got a collection of breakfast recipes that will get you started on the right foot every day, no matter how much or little time you have available for prep.

# Overnight Oats

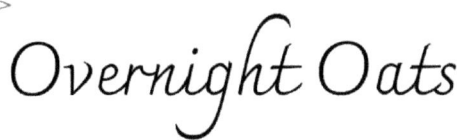

Overnight oats are a great choice to boost liver health and give yourself a carbohydrate boost to fuel you through the morning. But, since oats also have a ton of fiber in them, they are also great for digestion. By adding protein and some superfoods, you can get a perfect liver-friendly meal with almost no effort!
Here is how:

### INGREDIENTS

½ heaped cup of rolled oats
⅓ cup of plain Greek yogurt
⅓ cup of almond milk
Pinch of salt
Honey or maple syrup to taste

### OPTIONAL ADDITIONS

Chopped nuts (especially walnuts) or sunflower seeds
Chia seeds
Blueberries, cranberries or citrus fruits
Dark chocolate chips

### METHOD

Mix all ingredients together.
Spoon into a screw-top (mason) jar.
Refrigerate overnight.
Open, eat from the jar, and enjoy!

NOTES

# Huevos Rancheros

Eggs are a fantastic breakfast food, and because they are high in protein, they are also great for helping your liver repair and rebuild itself. Huevos rancheros is a classic Tex-Mex style dish, and we have lightened it up and added lots of liver-friendly ingredients to make it perfect for liver health!

## INGREDIENTS

Extra virgin olive oil for cooking vegetables and eggs
½ onion, chopped
1 tomato, peeled and coarsely chopped
½ cup black beans, drained and rinsed
Low sodium taco seasoning
1 egg
½ avocado, coarsely chopped
¼ cup plain Greek yogurt
Hot sauce (optional)

## METHOD

Soften the onion in olive oil.
Sprinkle in taco seasoning to taste and add roughly chopped tomatoes.
Cook over medium heat, stirring occasionally, until onions and tomatoes are soft.
Add beans to pan and heat through.
Keep vegetable mixture warm.
Fry egg to desired doneness.
Spoon vegetable mixture onto a plate and top with egg.
Add chopped avocados and yogurt and add hot sauce if using.

## NOTES

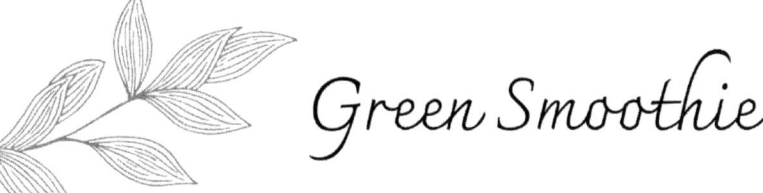

# Green Smoothie

Smoothies are a great choice when you are short on time, and you need breakfast you can enjoy on the run. This green smoothie packs a ton of liver healthy ingredients into one magical emerald package.

## INGREDIENTS

Frozen banana
Frozen mango or pineapple, or a combination of each
Spinach (baby spinach blends better!)
Romaine lettuce
Beet greens and carrot tops
Greek yogurt for added protein
Green tea to thin your smoothie
Honey

## METHOD

Add equal parts fruit and greens to the blender.
Blend until a smooth, thick mixture is achieved.
Add a drizzle of green tea and honey to taste.
Blend again to mix in tea and sweetener, then pour into a large glass or travel bottle, and enjoy!

# NOTES

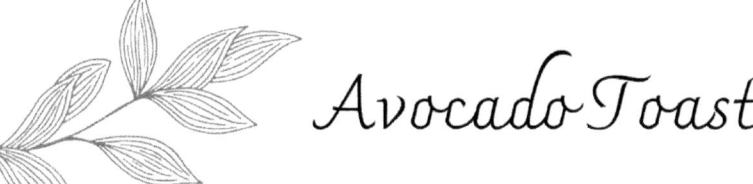

# Avocado Toast

Hey, it is trendy for a reason! Avocado toast is the perfect blend of healthy fats, whole grains, and tasty breakfast goodness!

## INGREDIENTS

2 slices natural whole grain bread, toasted
Avocado, mashed
Crushed garlic
Lemon juice
Salt and pepper to taste
Optional tomato slices

## METHOD

Mix the mashed avocado with the crushed garlic, lemon juice, and salt and pepper.
Spoon onto the whole-grain toast.
Top with tomato slices if using and enjoy!

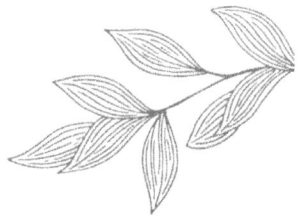

NOTES

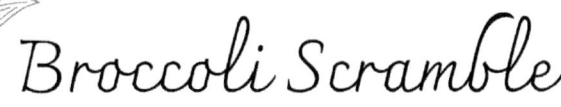

# Broccoli Scramble

In general, green foods are great for your liver, and broccoli is one of the best. This broccoli scramble is super easy to make, tastes great, and combines the antioxidants in broccoli with the lean protein in eggs.

### INGREDIENTS

1 or 2 crushed garlic cloves
Olive oil for sautéing
1 cup frozen broccoli
Two eggs, beaten with a little milk and seasoned to taste

### METHOD

Heat the oil in a pan over medium heat. (Do not get the pan sizzling hot, because olive oil cannot handle high heat, and garlic burns very easily!)
Sauté the garlic in the oil until slightly softened and fragrant. Add the frozen broccoli. Do not defrost first, the liquid from melting ice will help to ensure it cooks through. Stir fry until softened.
Pour eggs over softened broccoli and scramble.

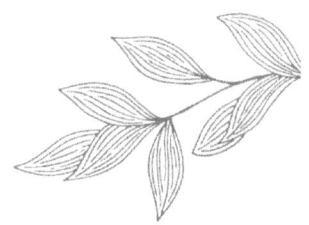

NOTES

# Fruit Parfait

Who does not love breakfast that looks like dessert? Even better when it is healthy, so you can feel good about it too!

### INGREDIENTS

Crushed nuts and sunflower seeds
Mixed fruit (berries are a great choice, but peaches, mango, and kiwi are also excellent choices) chopped
Plain Greek yogurt
Honey

### METHOD

Place a layer of crushed nuts and seeds at the bottom of a wide glass.
Add a layer of chopped fruit.
Spoon in a layer of plain yogurt.
Drizzle with honey, and then repeat layers, finishing with more honey and a final sprinkle of nuts.

NOTES

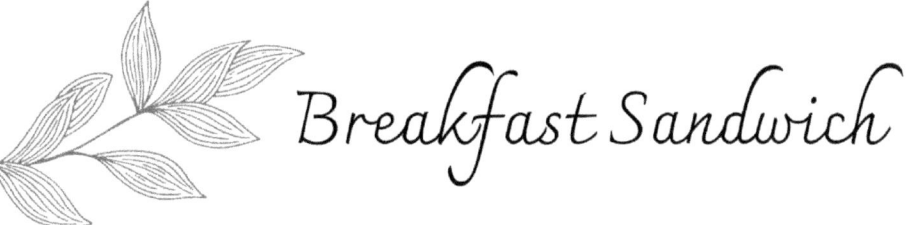

# Breakfast Sandwich

No, you cannot have a fast-food breakfast sandwich, but you can have the next best thing - a liver-friendly, veggie-heavy version!

## INGREDIENTS

Whole wheat English muffin
½ avocado mixed with lemon and salt and pepper
Sautéed spinach
1 poached egg
Dijon mustard

## METHOD

Cut the muffin in half, and spread one side with mashed avocado, and the other with a thin layer of mustard.
Add the poached egg.
Top with the sautéed spinach, close up your sandwich, and enjoy a lighter, liver healthy breakfast sandwich alternative!

# NOTES

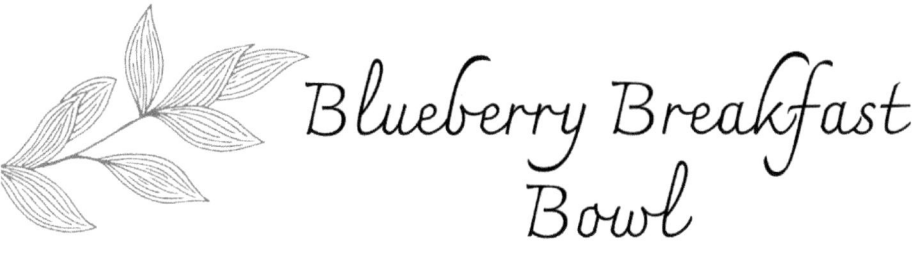

# Blueberry Breakfast Bowl

There is a good reason bowls are so popular these days - they are super easy to make and require fewer dishes! When you add tons of liver healthy ingredients, they are great for your health too.

## INGREDIENTS

2 ripe bananas
1 cup blueberries
1/2 cup almond milk
2 tsp coconut oil
2 tsp bee pollen or honey
1 tbsp almond butter
*To garnish*:
chia seeds crushed almonds, coconut flakes, bee pollen, more blueberries

## METHOD

Add all the ingredients to a blender.
Pulse until the desired smoothness is achieved.
Spoon into a bowl.
Top with your choice of garnishes for extra taste and crunch!

## NOTES

# Sweet Potato Pancakes

Who said liver healthy breakfast had to be boring? These sweet potato pancakes are so easy to make. Combine the fiber, vitamin C and beta carotene, and lean protein to help support and heal your liver.

## INGREDIENTS

1 medium sweet potato, baked, cooled, and peeled
2 large eggs
Cinnamon
Olive oil for pan
Honey to serve

## METHOD

Blend or process sweet potatoes and eggs with cinnamon to taste until smooth.
Drop spoonsful of the mixture into a hot pan that is lightly greased with olive oil.
Gently lift the edge of a pancake after a minute or two. The bottom will be golden brown when ready to flip, but the top will not bubble like your regular pancakes.
Flip onto other side when ready.
Serve hot pancakes with a drizzle of honey.

NOTES

# Easy Breakfast Frittata

Why waste time with fussy omelets when you can make a simple frittata packed with liver boosting vegetables!

## INGREDIENTS

One egg, beaten
Olive oil for pan
Plain Greek yogurt or low fat cottage cheese to serve

Choose two or more vegetables from the list below, for about a cup of chopped veggies in total:

- Tomatoes
- Onions
- Mushrooms
- Broccoli
- Spinach

## METHOD

Add a little olive oil to a small oven-safe skillet, and sauté gently over medium-high heat until just tender.
Whisk eggs with a tablespoon of water and season to taste.
Pour eggs into skillet and allow them to flow around the vegetables.
Leave the skillet on the stove for one or two minutes, until the bottom of the egg is set.
Transfer the skillet to the oven, and finish under the grill until the top of the egg is golden brown.
Serve with plain yogurt or low-fat cottage cheese.

NOTES

# LUNCH & DINNER

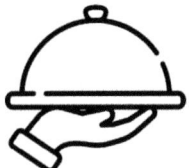

Lunch and dinner options when you are on a liver detox are incredibly varied. Base dishes on lean protein, plenty of healthy vegetables, and a small amount of whole grains, and you cannot go wrong. Because herbs and spices are so good for your liver, switch out your regular condiments for hot Mexican inspired spices, or warm Indian blends. Add lemon and lime juice for extra tang and switch out low-fat plain yogurt for cream sauces.

Here are a few great recipes you can use to get your liver detox started!

# Spaghetti Squash Marinara

It is comfort food that is also good for you. By swapping noodles for spaghetti squash, you can turn pasta into a liver-friendly meal that tastes great. Cooked tomatoes are a lot more bioavailable. A tiny sprinkling of good parmesan cheese improves flavor but is not necessary or particularly liver-friendly.

## INGREDIENTS

1 large can of chopped tomatoes (choose one that has no added salt)
½ onion, chopped
2 cloves garlic, crushed
1 tsp mixed herbs
Salt and pepper to taste
Olive oil
½ spaghetti squash
Sprinkling of parmesan cheese (optional)

## METHOD

Scoop the seeds out of the spaghetti squash, place cut side down on a baking sheet and bake in a 400F oven for 40 minutes or until soft. Remove and cool.
Heat olive oil in a heavy bottom saucepan, over a medium heat. Add onions and garlic and stir fry until softened. Do not allow to burn.
Add herbs, salt, and pepper, and then add the can of tomatoes, along with about a cup of water.
Simmer for 30-40 minutes, or until the tomatoes are soft and the water has boiled away. Taste and adjust seasoning.
Scrape squash out of skins and place in a bowl. Top with marinara sauce and add a sprinkling of cheese for flavor.

NOTES

# Moroccan Chicken with Chickpeas and Quinoa

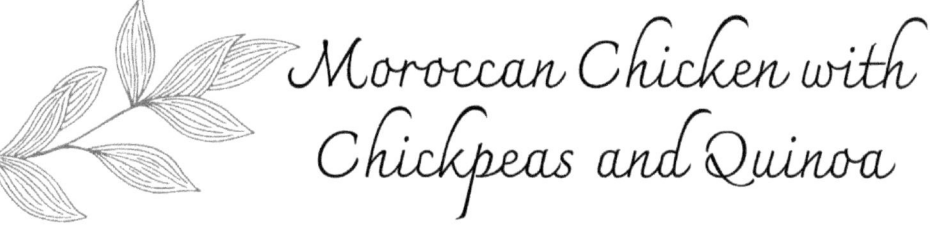

Turmeric and other spices are great for liver health, as are whole grains, vegetables, and legumes. This easy dish combines all the absolute best foods for your liver into one delicious package.

## INGREDIENTS

1 Boneless, skinless chicken breast, cut into strips
½ tsp each turmeric, chili flakes, cumin, and parsley
1 clove garlic, crushed
Squeeze of lemon
2 tbsp plain yogurt
Salt and pepper to taste
Olive oil for skillet
1 cup cooked quinoa
½ cup finely chopped tomatoes
½ cup finely chopped cucumber
½ cup canned chickpeas, drained and rinsed
¼ cup orange juice
1 tsp hot sauce

## METHOD

Mix herbs and spices with garlic, lemon, and yogurt.
Coat chicken strips in marinade mixture and allow to sit for about ten minutes.
Heat a ridged skillet and grill the chicken until cooked through and marked on both sides. Set aside.
Mix the orange juice and hot sauce, and stir into quinoa, chickpeas, and vegetables.
Top quinoa mixture with grilled chicken.

NOTES

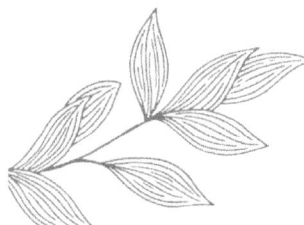

# Sweet Potato Spinach Curry

Curry is an excellent dish for liver health, especially if it is made with vegetables and lean protein. This simple vegetarian curry combines warm spices with creamy yogurt. When served over brown rice, it is a hearty lunch or supper dish.

## INGREDIENTS

½ onion, chopped
2 cloves garlic
1 - 2 tsp curry powder (depending on strength and personal taste)
½ tsp each chili flakes, cumin, cardamom and turmeric
Salt and pepper to taste
1 tomato, peeled, seeded and chopped
1 medium sweet potato, peeled and cut into 1" chunks
2 cups baby spinach, washed
½ cup plain Greek yogurt
1 cup cooked brown rice to serve

## METHOD

Sauté onion and garlic until translucent.
Add spices, salt and pepper to pan and fry until fragrant.
Add chopped tomatoes and a little water and cook until water is nearly evaporated, and the mixture has thickened slightly.
Add sweet potatoes and cook until nearly soft.
Add spinach and wilt, then stir in yogurt, and adjust seasoning.
Serve over brown rice.

# NOTES

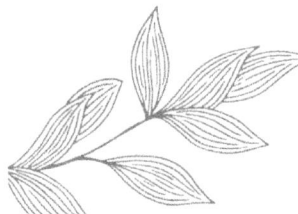

# Teriyaki Salmon and Crunchy Green Salad

Oily fish like salmon has healthy fat and lean protein, which makes it great for your liver and for your health in general. Vegetables and fruit all have phytochemicals, vitamins, and antioxidants that we need to stay healthy. This meal combines it all in one tasty package.

## INGREDIENTS

Salmon filet
¼ cup low salt soy sauce
2 tbsp honey
Olive oil
Salad greens (any or all of kale, spinach, lettuce, and dandelion greens)
Tart green apple, cut into wedges
Walnuts, chopped
½ onion, slivered
1 tbsp honey
Lemon juice
Salt and pepper to taste

## METHOD

Mix soy sauce and honey together.
Heat oil in a pan, and place the salmon, skin side down, in the pan.
Cook for a few minutes on the skin side, and then turn to finish.
Assemble the salad ingredients.
Mix honey, lemon juice, and seasoning together and dress salad with a drizzle.
Place salmon on a plate, and drizzle with teriyaki sauce.

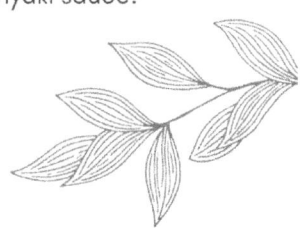

## NOTES

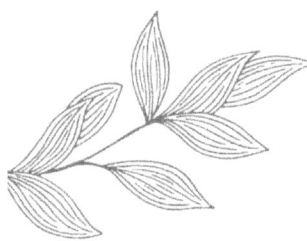

# Hearty Vegetable Soup

Vegetables are great for your liver, and soup is a great way to cook them because all the nutrients that come out during the cooking process stay in the broth.

## INGREDIENTS

½ chopped onion
2 - 3 stalks of celery, chopped
1 large carrot, scrubbed and chopped
1 small potato, peeled and chopped
1 peeled and chopped tomato
1 diced zucchini
1 small can kidney beans, drained and rinsed
2 cloves of garlic, crushed
1 tsp mixed herbs
½ cup uncooked barley
Salt and pepper to taste
Low salt or homemade vegetable stock
Olive oil
Whole-grain toast, to serve

## METHOD

Heat olive oil in a medium-sized saucepan.
Add onions, carrots, and celery, and stir fry over medium heat until translucent.
Add the remainder of vegetables, barley, herbs, and stock to saucepan.
Stir, cover and simmer for 30 to 45 minutes, or until vegetables are tender and barley is cooked through.
Adjust seasoning and serve with whole-grain toast.

# NOTES

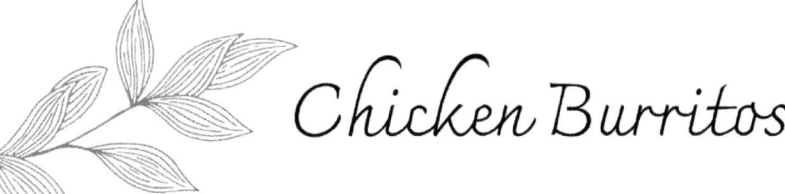

# Chicken Burritos

Burritos are actually a surprisingly healthy and liver-friendly meal when made at home. These tasty burritos are made with whole-grain tortillas and packed with lean protein and delicious vegetables.

## INGREDIENTS

1 boneless, skinless chicken breast
Reduced salt taco seasoning
Olive oil
Chopped tomatoes
Chopped red onions
Chopped avocados
Shredded cabbage
Chopped coriander / cilantro (optional)
Lime wedges
Plain Greek yogurt
Hot sauce to taste

## METHOD

Heat olive oil in a medium-sized saucepan.
Add chicken and brown on all sides.
Add about a cup of water and taco seasoning and poach chicken until cooked through. Remove chicken from heat and cool.
Shred chicken, then build burritos with vegetables of your choice, shredded chicken, yogurt, lime juice, and hot sauce.

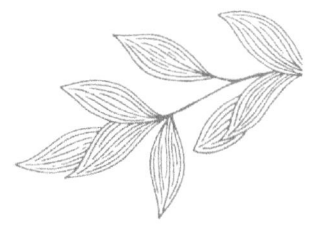

## NOTES

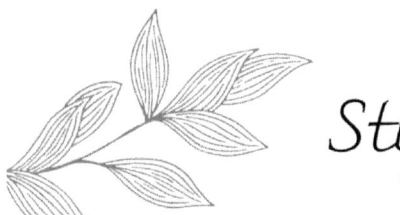

# Stuffed Peppers

Sweet peppers are packed with vitamin C and other liver healthy minerals and vitamins. When they are stuffed with lean meat, tasty vegetables, and other tasty goodies and baked, they make an easy and delicious meal.

## INGREDIENTS

1 sweet bell pepper (recipe is per person, multiply accordingly)
¼ lb. lean ground turkey, pork or chicken per person
¼ finely chopped onion
Olive oil for sautéing
¼ cup chopped mushrooms
½ chopped zucchini
½ cup diced mixed peppers
¼ cup spinach
1 peeled and seeded tomato, finely chopped
1 crushed garlic clove
1 tsp mixed herbs
Salt and pepper to taste
Plain low-fat cottage cheese to serve

## METHOD

Preheat oven to 350F.
Cut the top off the pepper and remove the core.
Heat olive oil in a medium-sized saucepan.
Add ground meat to pan, breaking up as you brown it. Add salt and pepper to taste.
Add onion to browned meat, and sauté till starting to become translucent.
Add remaining vegetables and spices and cook until vegetables are softened, and most of the liquid has evaporated.
Stuff meat and vegetable mixture into pepper, top with cottage cheese, and place stuffed pepper into a ramekin, with a small amount of water around the pepper.
Place pepper into the oven and bake until the flesh of the pepper has softened, and the cottage cheese is lightly browned. Serve.

NOTES

# Cauliflower Buffalo "Wings"

Yes, sometimes you want something spicy and delicious. These cauliflower buffalo "wings" are just the thing, and if you serve them with sweet potato oven wedges on the side, you've got the ideal liver-friendly "cheat" meal!

## INGREDIENTS

½ a head of cauliflower, cut into florets
¼ cup natural almond milk
¼ cup water
½ cup all-purpose flour
1 tsp garlic powder
1 tsp onion powder
½ tsp each cumin and paprika
Salt and pepper to taste
Celery sticks to serve
Sweet potato wedges to serve
Plain yogurt to serve
Buffalo sauce to serve

## METHOD

Preheat oven to 450F.
Mix dry ingredients together.
Mix water and almond milk.
Dip florets into almond milk, then dredge. Repeat, and place coated florets on a baking sheet.
Bake for 15 minutes, then flip and bake another 10 minutes on the other side.
Remove the florets from the oven, and coat in buffalo sauce.
Serve "wings" with sweet potato fries, celery sticks, more buffalo sauce for dipping, and plain yogurt for dipping.

## NOTES

# Portobello Mushroom Burgers

When you switch out the meat for mushroom, a juicy burger can be a liver-friendly treat!

## INGREDIENTS

1 large portobello mushroom, stem removed
Garlic
Olive oil
Salt and pepper to taste
1 tsp mixed herbs
¼ cup water
Plain yogurt
Sliced tomato
Lettuce leaves
Dijon mustard
Plain cottage cheese
Whole grain burger buns
Sweet potato fries to serve

## METHOD

Heat oil in a frying pan.
Season mushroom with salt and pepper and herbs, and add to pan, cap side down.
Pour water around the mushroom cap, so that it steams lightly before it fries.
Flip mushroom over to cook other side.
Cut bun in half and spread with a mixture of yogurt and Dijon mustard.
Layer vegetables on bun.
Remove mushroom from pan and fill the "cavity" under the cap with cottage cheese.
Serve with sweet potato fries.

# NOTES

# SNACKS

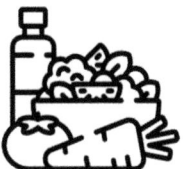

Because your liver is so closely tied to other systems and organs, like your pancreas, and because it's so involved in processing sugar and carbohydrates, it's smart to take a trick out of the diabetes diet cookbook. This means making sure that your snacks balance carbohydrates and protein with some healthy fat. This helps to ensure that there is less spike in your blood sugar and less strain on your system as it tries to cope.

This table is designed to give you *mix and match* snack options that make it easy to find the perfect combo!

| CARBOHYDRATE | PROTEIN |
| --- | --- |
| Apple | Peanut butter & celery |
| 3 whole grain crackers | Slice of low fat cheddar |
| ½ handful of raisins | Cottage cheese |
| ½ slice wholegrain toast | ½ handful of almonds |
| ½ cup natural trail mix | ½ avocado |
| Orange | Boiled egg |
| Banana | Slice of roast chicken |
| Oven baked sweet potato | Hummus & veggies |
| Lentils or oatmeal | Edamame |

Other great snack choices include a few squares of dark chocolate with some fresh berries or a few root vegetable chips with homemade hummus.

The key to healthy snacking is moderation and balance. Carbs on their own are a bad idea, but when they are combined with protein and a little bit of healthy fat, they will fill you up and fuel you at the same time. That's good for your liver and your waistline!

# JUICES & SHAKES

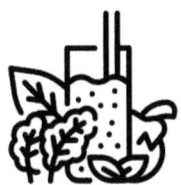

J uices are a great way to get a lot of nutrition in a quick and convenient package. However, always remember that when it comes to juices, shakes, and smoothies, the fresher, the better, so make them at home. That way, you can also control the addition of sugar and other not so great ingredients. Here are some simple and easy to make juices, shakes, and smoothies for you to try.

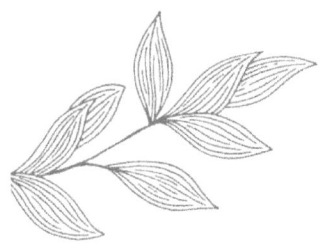

# *Juices*

### CARROT & ORANGE

Juice one orange and one carrot

### APPLE, GINGER & KALE

Juice one apple, one cup of spinach and about half an inch of fresh ginger

### CRANBERRY BEET

Juice one small red beetroot with a cup of cranberries, and add a little honey to sweeten

### POMEGRANATE GREEN TEA

Equal parts pomegranate and green tea, sweetened with honey

### VIRGIN MARY

Juice tomatoes with celery, add lemon juice and a shot of hot sauce

### PINA-BANANA-COLADA

Juice a cup of pineapple chunks, one banana and a cup of coconut water

### CUCUMBER, APPLE & CELERY

Juice one apple, a couple of sticks of celery, and a 2-3" chunk of cucumber

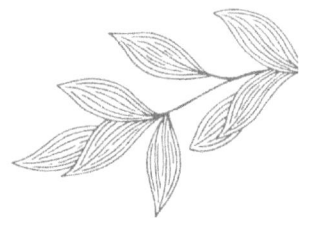

## NOTES

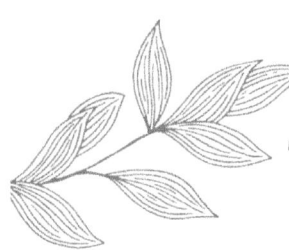

# Smoothies and Shakes

## STRAW-NANA

Blend a cup of strawberries with one banana, thin with freshly squeezed orange juice, and add ½ a cup of plain low-fat Greek yogurt.

## CHOCO-NUT

Blend 1 cup plain unsweetened almond milk with 2 tablespoons of almond butter and one banana, add 1 tablespoon of coco powder and sweeten to taste with honey or stevia.

## GREEN & MEAN

Blend one kiwi fruit, a cup of spinach, a cup of pineapple, one banana, and a cup of orange juice to thin the mixture.

## PEACH-MANGO-TURMERIC

Blend 1 cup peaches, 1 cup mango, and one banana. Thin with orange juice and add ¼ teaspoon each of turmeric and ginger.

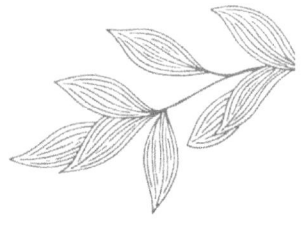

# NOTES

Nearly any combination of fruits and vegetables can be used to make powerhouse liver-friendly shakes and smoothies. Adding nut butter or plain yogurt adds a little protein to make them a full meal on their own.

When you want to thin smoothies or juices, freshly squeezed juices or green tea are fantastic options, and you can use honey, maple syrup, or stevia if you need a little sweetness.

Smoothies and shakes are a great way to add more healthy spices to your diet. Turmeric, cinnamon, and ginger are all great additions.

When you have any doubt about what to drink, the best choice for a thirst quencher is always water, possibly with a little lemon. Enough water is critical to the health of your liver, and everything else in your body.

# 7 DAY MEAL PLAN

As you can see, there are plenty of great-tasting, healthy foods you can choose to boost your overall health and support your liver's oh so important role in your body. But to make it even simpler, we have devised a 7-day sample menu using variations on these recipes and other simple foods, so you can kickstart your new eating plan without breaking a sweat.

Feel free to switch out any of the recipes and gain further inspiration from the recipes listed before.

# Sample 7 Day Meal Plan

| DAY | BREAKFAST | LUNCH | DINNER |
| --- | --- | --- | --- |
| Monday | Overnight Oats | Avocado Toast | Broccoli scramble |
| Tuesday | Wholegrain toast with low fat cottage cheese & tomato | Moroccan Chicken & Quinoa | Sweet potato spinich curry |
| Wednesday | Half a wholegrain bagel with 1 scrambled egg | Teriyaki Salmon Salad | Stuffed peppers |
| Thursday | English muffin with avocado & tomato | Spagetti squash | Chicken burritos |
| Friday | Breakfast frittata | Avocado Toast | Cauliflower buffalo wings |
| Saturday | Blueberry breakfast bowl | Stuffed peppers | Portobello mushroom burger |
| Sunday | Fruit parfait | Whole grain pita with garlic hummus | Vegetable soup |

### OPTIONAL SNACK

*Feel free to add a daily snack from our snacks chart.

Each of these dinner menus could be finished with a small bowl of fresh fruit or berries, a small spoon of low-fat plain yogurt, and a drizzle of honey.

It does not have to be hard to eat well or boring. With a menu like this, and a few more vegetable-heavy, liver healthy dishes in your repertoire, you can eat very well every day, and still do great things for your health!

**Food Is More Than Just Fuel**

You may have read this chapter thinking that the recipes do not sound bad, and the diet does not look too hard to stick to, and that is true. Food doesn't have to taste bad to be good for you. By making small tweaks and smart substitutions, you can eat delicious food, be healthier, and take better care of your liver (and the rest of your organs!)

Food contains so many chemicals and compounds, good and bad, that we can use to improve our health, immune system and heal our organs.

The food we eat can support traditional medical treatments for conditions we are diagnosed with, but it can also help us have more energy, lose weight easier, and fuel us when we exercise.

We hope that reading how easy it can be to make better food choices every day helps inspire you to try it. If you do, remember that as long as you make good choices 90% of the time, you can get away with cheating the other 10%. The world will not end if you have some pizza or a cookie but follow it with a juice or a vegetarian meal choice.

Food alone cannot give you perfect health, however. You need a few more things, like exercise, which brings us to the end of the chapter, and the start of the next.

> While detox diets don't do anything that your body can't naturally do on its own, you can optimize your body's natural detoxification system.

―――――――――――――

*Healthline*

# 4

# SHAKE WHAT YOUR MAMA GAVE YOU!

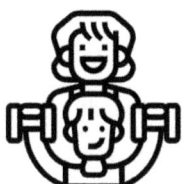

*"Good things come to those who sweat."*

I t is an old saying, but it is also true.

While fueling our body with the right things is a big part of overall health, and liver health in particular, exercise is also critical to our overall wellbeing. In fact, if you combine healthy eating with even moderate exercise, you can supercharge your liver and get all the benefits that come with that.

Exercise helps to get your blood flowing, has been proven to improve mental health, improves digestion, increases metabolism, and can even positively impact diabetes, among many other benefits. It is one of the best things you can do for yourself.

But exercise does not have to be difficult, expensive, or boring.

If you hate aerobics classes, do not do them. If gyms make you yawn, avoid them.

You do not even have to get out of your pajamas to exercise (although it will be more comfortable if you do!)

How Exercise Helps Your Liver

We all know that in general, exercise is a good idea, and we have already mentioned some of the more impressive benefits you will see if you start exercising regularly. But exercise also has very specific benefits for your liver. These include:

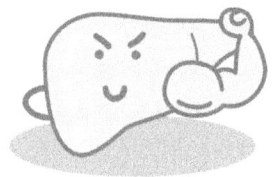

- Weight loss. When you exercise regularly and eat healthily, you will lose weight. Since carrying excess weight is a risk factor for fatty liver disease, that gives you a better chance to either avoid it or limit its impact.
- Research has shown, in fact, that exercise is a key factor in reducing hepatic fat. This fat is specific to your liver. Studies have even shown that you do not have to see external weight loss to get a significant benefit from even half an hour of exercise every other day.
- Exercise also has a positive impact on insulin resistance, which is proven in studies involving diabetics. Since your liver is intimately involved in the storage and release of sugar, it is excellent for your liver.
- Exercise improves circulation. Since your liver is an organ that is an integral part of the circulatory system, getting blood

- flowing through it faster and more efficiently can have major benefits.
- Exercise also helps you to sweat, and sweating is another way to excrete toxins from your body. Fewer toxins, of course, mean a happier liver.
- Exercise has even been proven, in studies, to protect your liver from alcohol-related damage.
- Finally, because exercise improves mental health, you are less likely to turn to unhealthy choices. This means you will be less likely to binge eat, drink alcohol, and smoke to boost your mood. This is always good news for your liver!

You do not have to spend hours in the gym to get these benefits either.

A brisk walk around a neighborhood park with your dog, or half an hour on an exercise bike while you watch your favorite show a few times a week are all it takes to get enough exercise to start seeing health benefits.

It does not matter what you do to burn energy – whether it is tobogganing with your kids or mowing the lawn. It all counts, and the more you do, the better for your body and your liver.

Yoga

Yoga is a great practice to include in your weekly health routine. It can be particularly helpful in improving liver health. This is because yoga is not only excellent for its fitness aspects but also incorporates breathing and elements of "*finding your calm*". It can help you both de-stress and get in great shape. With the body control you gain, you will feel ready to conquer the world.

We wanted to add some simple poses and stretches you can perform to get a small taste of yoga. As an added benefit, these poses are said to help detoxify your liver.

Make sure not to push your body past any point you aren't comfortable with.

# Seated Twist

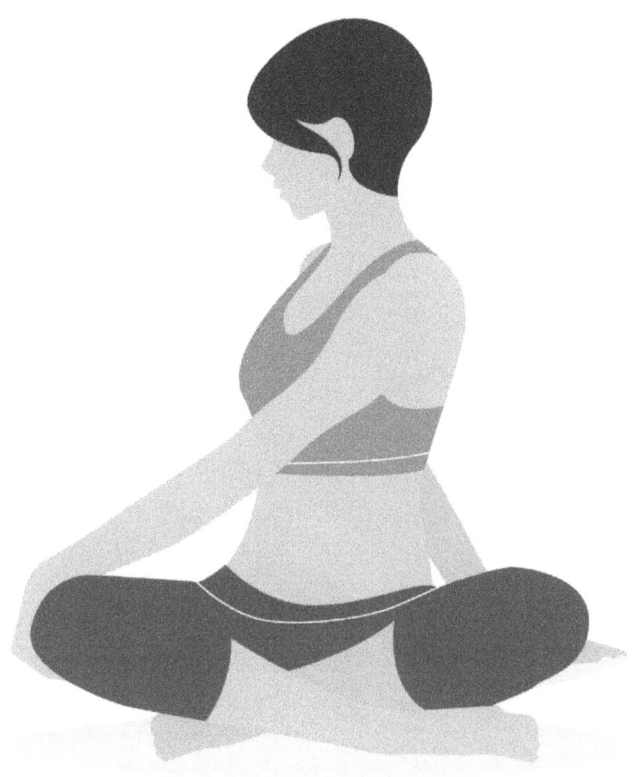

Get in a comfortable cross-legged seated position. Aim to sit with a tall spine and engaged core. With a deep inhale, raise your arms and lengthen your spine. On your exhale, slowly twist your upper body towards the right and look over your right shoulder. Place your right hand behind you and your left hand on your right knee. Stay in this pose for 5 to 10 breaths. Optionally and, if possible, lightly deepen your twist with each exhale. Once complete, repeat on the other side.

# Side Body Stretch

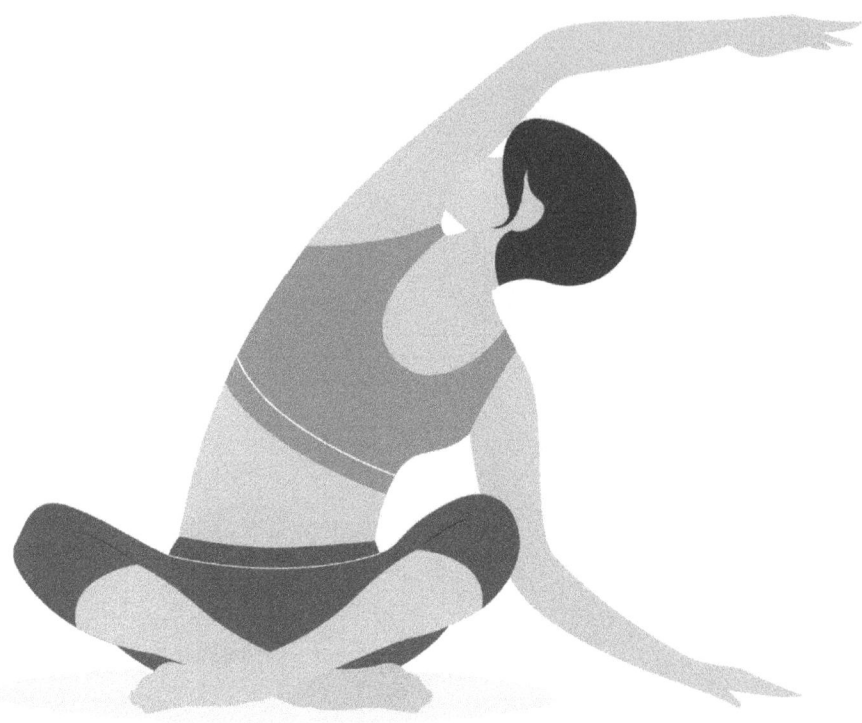

Start in a comfortable cross-legged seated position. Aim to sit with a tall spine and engaged core. With a deep inhale, raise your arms and lengthen your spine. On your exhale, place your left arm to your left side and shift your right arm and upper body to the left. Simultaneously shift your gaze upwards. Stay in this pose for 5 to 10 breaths. Once complete, repeat on the other side.

# Thread the Needle

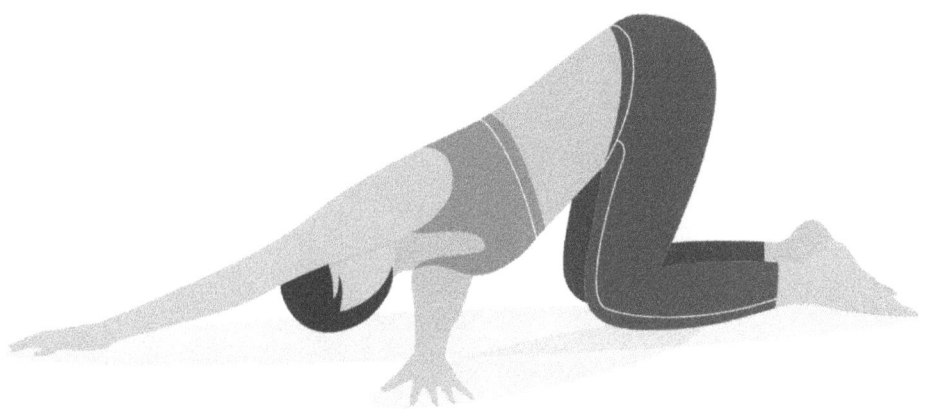

Get on your hands and knees, both shoulder and hip apart. Inhale. On your exhale, reach your right arm under your left arm. Continue by lowering your right shoulder and ear to your mat. Keep your hips in the air and maintain an equal weight in your knees. Hold this pose for 5 to 10 breaths. Once complete, release back to a neutral position on your hands and knees. Then repeat on the other side.

# Revolved Chair

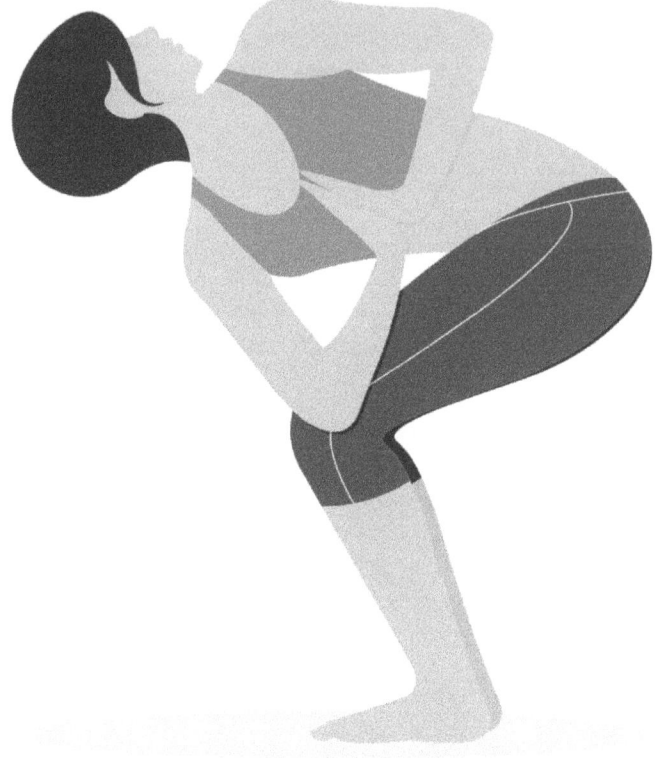

Stand straight up with your chest out and feet and knees together. As you inhale, raise your arms overhead with your palms facing each other. Place your weight mostly on your heels, and as you exhale, bend your knees and lower yourself down as if you were to sit on a chair. As you inhale, lower your hands down to your chest palms coming together in a prayer position. Then as you exhale, twist your chest and shoulders towards the right and aim to place your right elbow outside of your left leg. Try to hold this pose for 5 to 10 breaths before slowly releasing and returning to a relaxed straight-up stance. Repeat on the other side.

# Warrior 1

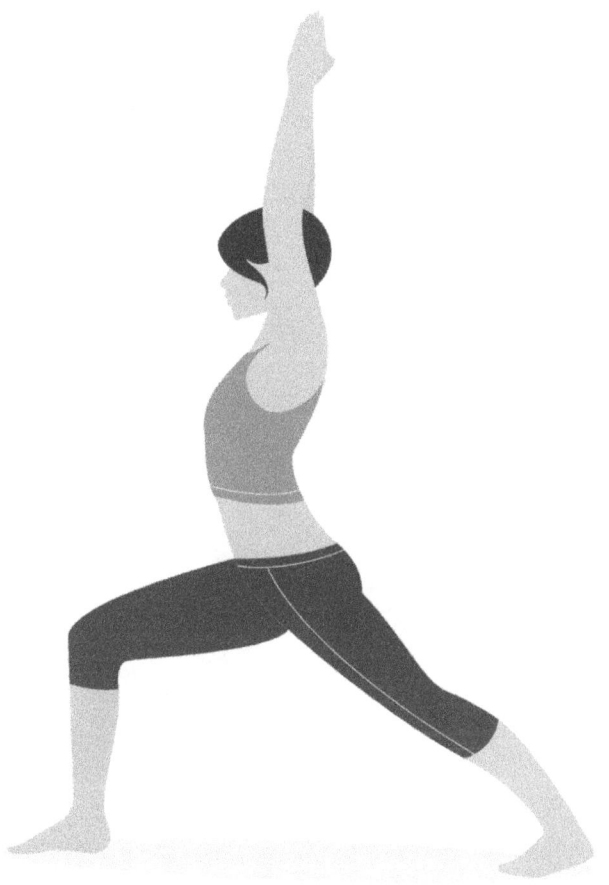

Begin by stepping your right foot forward and pointing your feet straight ahead. Your chest and belly button should also point forward. Keep your left leg behind you and turn your heel inward, making your left toes point outward at about a 45-degree angle. On an inhale, raise your arms straight above your head with your palms facing one another. Focus on lifting your chest and keeping your core tight. Hold this pose for 5 to 10 breaths. Repeat with your left leg forward and right leg back.

# Reverse Warrior

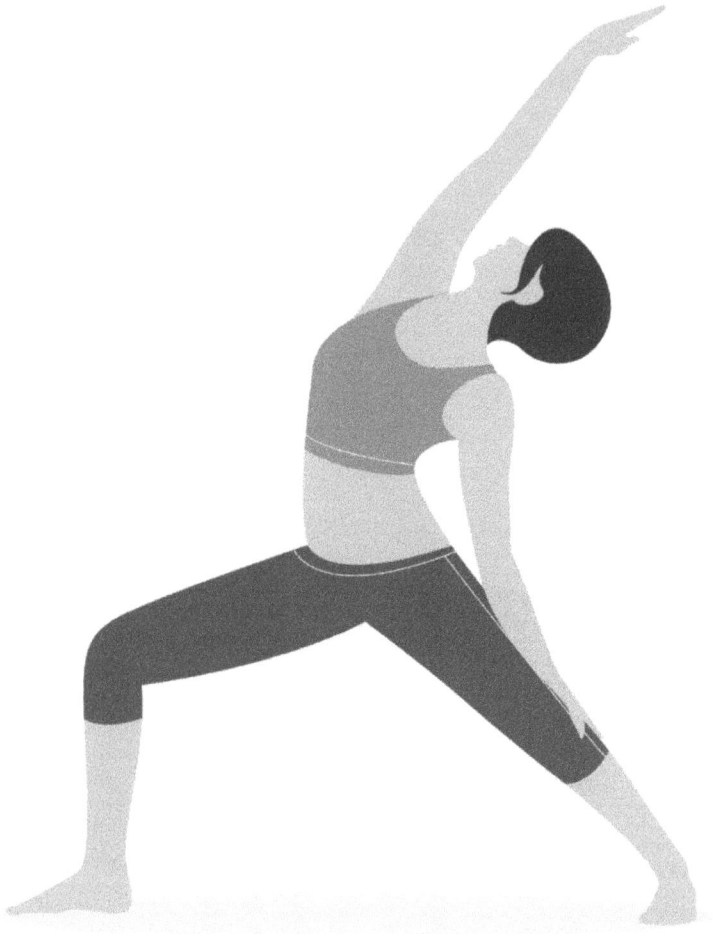

From Warrior 1, lower your arms inline with your shoulders and twist your chest and belly button inward. Lower your left arm and let it rest on your left leg. Inhale and bring your right arm up and to the back. Look up, so you don't place too much strain on your neck. Hold this pose for 3 to 8 breaths. Slowly release back to a neutral position and repeat on the other side.

# Warrior Twist

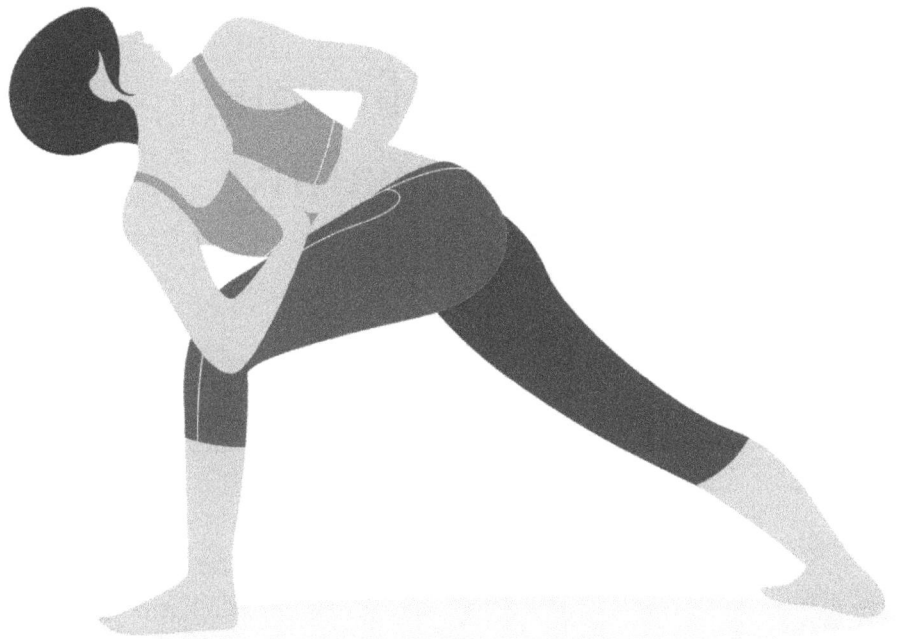

From warrior 1, on an inhale, bring your palms together on your chest. As you exhale, twist your torso towards your leading leg. Following the diagram above, it is the left leg. Aim to place your elbow on the outside of the leading leg. Turn your face to look upwards, unless this is uncomfortable. Hold this pose for 3 to 8 breaths. Slowly release to a neutral position and repeat on the other side.

**66**

Love yourself enough
to live a healthy
lifestyle

---

*Jules Robson*

# AFTERWORD

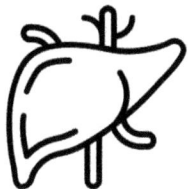

We started this book by introducing you to the unsung hero that is your liver. You learned how important your liver is in nearly everything your body does, and why, when your liver is not performing at its peak, it can affect all kinds of things in your life.

Along the way, we looked at some potentially serious liver conditions, which you hopefully don't have yet. We showed you how to avoid them, and how to potentially roll back damage you might have unknowingly done to your liver before you read this book.

Perhaps most importantly, though, we hope we showed you how a large part of your liver health is directly related to what you eat, drink, and do in your life. But also, because your liver is the only organ you have that can heal itself, you have the time to change your liver health.

While you might not be able to avoid all of the diseases, disorders, and conditions that might affect your liver, you do hold all the power to stop overworking your liver and start fueling it and giving it the nutrients it needs to do its essential work.

Your liver is central to so many things in your body that we can almost guarantee that if you make the simple changes we outline in this book, you will feel better, look better, and live a happier, healthier life.

Because your liver might not be the flashiest organ you have, but it is one of the most important, and you owe it to yourself to take care of it.

> If you don't take care of this the most magnificent machine that you will ever be given...where are you going to live?

— Karyn Calabrese

## THANK YOU

Thank you for reading this book and allowing us to share our knowledge with you.

If you've enjoyed this book, please let us know by leaving an Amazon rating and a brief review! It only takes about 30 seconds, and it helps us compete against big publishing houses. It also helps other readers find my work!

Thank you for your time, and have an awesome day!

A healthy outside
starts from the inside.

*Robert Urich*

# RESOURCES

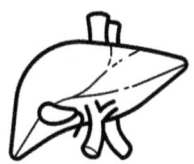

We have used many resources to compile the information in this book. While we hope we've taught you enough about your liver to make keeping it healthier easy, we know that you still might want to do a little more research. So, we have compiled a list of great liver resources you can visit and read to find out more.

**The Canadian Liver Foundation**

https://www.liver.ca/

The Canadian Liver Foundation is a non-profit organization devoted to all things liver health-related. Their website contains a wealth of information, including links to the most recent resources and research paper.

**The American Liver Foundation**

https://liverfoundation.org/

The American Liver Foundation is another well-conceived and comprehensive liver health resource. The glossary of liver diseases on the website is particularly useful if you are trying to make sense of a liver disease diagnosis.

**Hepatitis Foundation International**

https://hepatitisfoundation.org/

It may not be the best-looking website out there. Still, the Hepatitis Foundation International website is an invaluable resource for anyone looking to learn more about this family of liver conditions.

**Fatty Liver Foundation**

https://www.fattyliverfoundation.org

Learn more about the different kinds of fatty liver disease, treatment options, and how to live with fatty liver disease.

**Hepatitis Pages on the CDC website**

https://www.cdc.gov/hepatitis/hcv/cfaq.htm

The US Centers for Disease Control website has up to the minute research and information about all types of hepatitis. It is an excellent resource for prevention and treatment.

**British Liver Trust**

https://britishlivertrust.org.uk/information-and-support/living-with-a-liver-condition/diet-and-liver-disease/

The British Liver Trust website has a fantastic section about diet as a treatment and preventative measure for liver disease.

**Gastroenterology Center of Connecticut**

https://www.gastrocenter.org/our-centers/liver-center-at-gcc/diet-in-liver-disease/

Another fantastic resource for liver healthy diet advice.

**Hepatitis B Foundation**

https://www.hepb.org/

**Hepatitis C Association**

https://www.hepcassoc.org/

**Autoimmune Hepatitis Association**

https://www.aihep.org/

**Research Papers and Articles**

**What to do about non-alcoholic fatty liver disease**

https://www.health.harvard.edu/diseases-and-conditions/what-to-do-about-nonalcoholic-fatty-liver-disease

**High Intrinsic Aerobic Capacity Protects against Ethanol-Induced Hepatic Injury and Metabolic Dysfunction: Study Using High Capacity Runner Rat Model**

https://www.mdpi.com/2218-273X/5/4/3295

**Alcohol, liver, and nutrition.**

https://www.tandfonline.com/doi/abs/10.1080/07315724.1991.10718182

**Nutrition and survival in patients with liver cirrhosis**

https://www.sciencedirect.com/science/article/abs/pii/S0899900701005214

**Abundance of fructose not good for the liver, heart**

https://www.health.harvard.edu/heart-health/abundance-of-fructose-not-good-for-the-liver-heart

**Is your liver at risk?**

https://www.health.harvard.edu/diseases-and-conditions/is-your-liver-at-risk

**Fatigue in chronic liver disease: New insights and therapeutic approaches**

https://onlinelibrary.wiley.com/doi/full/10.1111/liv.13919

**Gender and racial differences in non-alcoholic fatty liver disease**

https://www.ncbi.nlm.nih.gov/pmc/articles/PMC4033285/

## OTHER BOOKS BY BRITTNEY & CRAIG

- Gut Detox & Cleanse

To find more of our books simply search or click our names on www.amazon.com

Milton Keynes UK
Ingram Content Group UK Ltd.
UKHW051256160624
444282UK00004B/15